Sea Sick

The Adventures of a Ship's Doctor

Sea
Sick

The Adventures of a Ship's Doctor

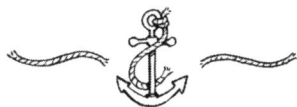

RUTH TAYLOR

T

Troubador Publishing Ltd
Unit E2 Airfield Business Park,
Harrison Road, Market Harborough,
Leicestershire. LE16 7UL
Tel: 0116 2792299
Email: books@troubador.co.uk
Web: www.troubador.co.uk

ISBN 978 1 80514 226 3

British Library Cataloguing in Publication Data.
A catalogue record for this book is available from the British Library.

Printed and bound in Great Britain by 4edge Limited
Typeset in 11pt Minion Pro by Troubador Publishing Ltd, Leicester, UK

To Tom

S.S. Sea Rainbow

Itinerary

Day 1	Southampton
Day 4	Madeira
Day 6	Tenerife
Day 10	Cape Verde Islands
Day 16	Fortaleza, Brazil
Day 17	Salvador, Brazil
Day 20	Rio de Janeiro, Brazil
Day 21	Rio to London Heathrow

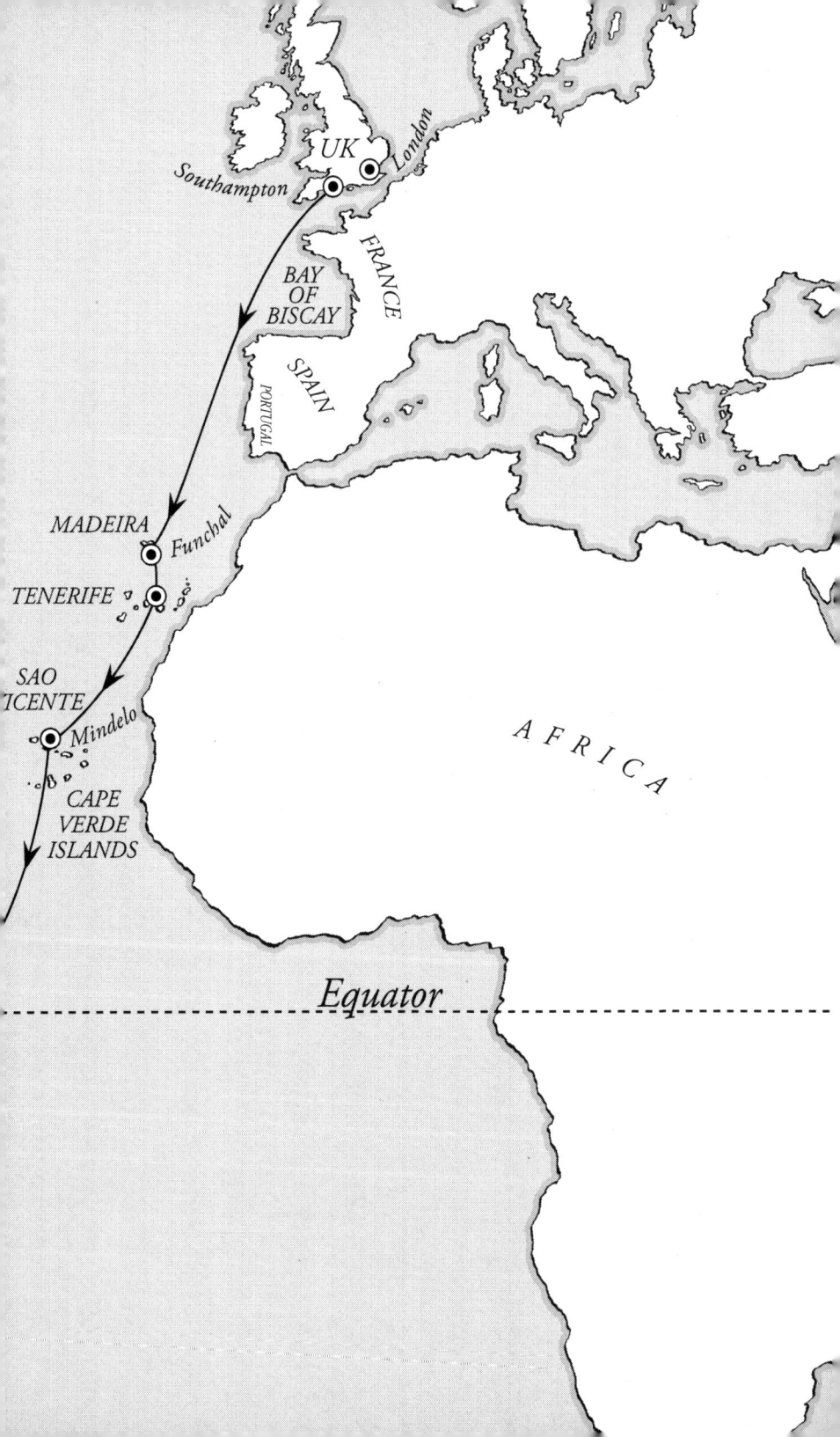

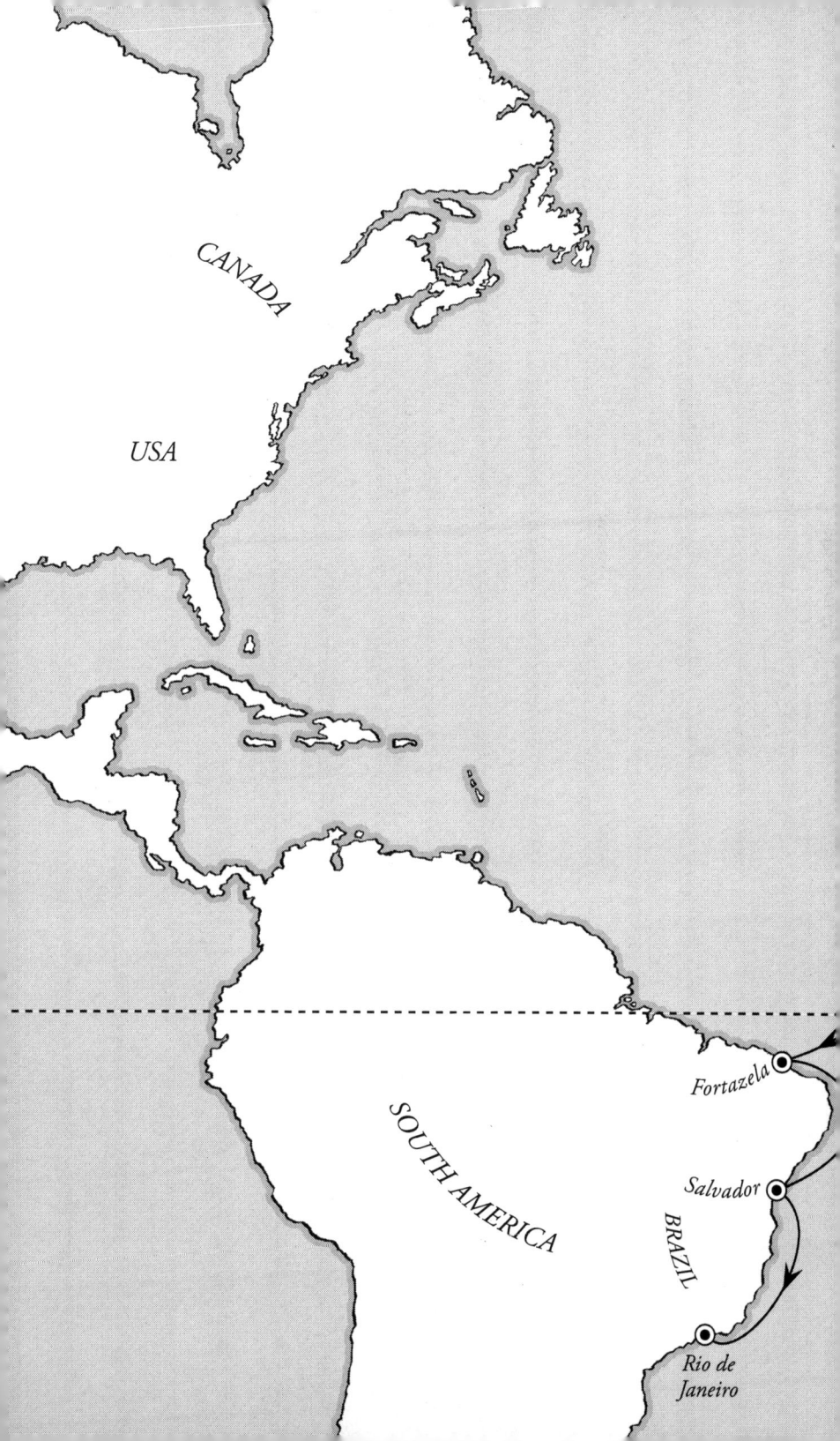

CANADA

USA

SOUTH AMERICA

BRAZIL

Fortazela

Salvador

Rio de
Janeiro

S.S. Sea Rainbow

Crew

Alberto – boatswain

Angel – receptionist

Anjan Shakya – deck-hand; arc eye

Anton – Second Engineer

Arvin Matapang – Maître d'

Brian – tall dance host

Captain Ivor Strom – Master

Cheryl – entertainments officer

The Confections: Carrie and Dave – vocalist and guitar duo

Coralie – nurse

Danang and Manas – waiters at Doctor's Table

Dayap – tailor

Dr Donald Wallis – Medical Director

Edward – younger dance host

Eric West – Cruise Director

Gabriel – laundry manager

Gary Pearce – stores manager

Jesus – galley hand

Joramae – reception manager

Joseph – port agent, Mindelo
Dr Katerina Klaus – helicopter rescue doctor
Kikato Mendoza – Security Officer
Lee Marsden – singer
Lenz Burger – head chef
Lisa – accountant
Liz – nurse
Lorenz – bar staff
Magic Moll – magician, comedienne
Mandy – dancer
Marcus Estaban – port agent, Tenerife
Mario – Sanitation Officer
Marion – shop manager
Mohan – Deputy Maître d'
Oleg Sotirov – Hotel Manager
Peter – older, slim dance host
Ramon Santos – Safety Officer
Rosa – stewardess
Sergei Kolomnikov – Chief Engineer
Tallak Steensen – Chief Officer
Zack – IT Officer

Passengers

Mr Albert Armsure – gastro. Wife, Edith, deceased
Alice – heart condition; Code Alpha
Barbara – friend of Pat; liaison with Reg
Baron Wild – cabaret singer
Dick – champion table tennis player; liaison with Mrs Plummer
Eleanor – single; engineer; usually with dance hosts
Mr Gardner – swollen legs; diabetic; dances with doctor
Mr Harold Olroyd – cabin companion to Albert Armsure, in an inside cabin
Jim & Mary – older couple at Doctor's Table
Mr John Richardson – pneumonia. Wife, Vera
Joyce & Len – quiz fans; friends of Derek & Pam
Mr Langford – high INR (thin blood)
Lesley – widow; often with dance hosts
Mr Marquez – cardiac arrest. Wife, Ana
Pam & Derek – younger married couple at Doctor's Table
Pat – allergic reaction; friend of Alice
Mrs Plummer – venereal condition. Husband, Arthur, liaison with Magic Moll
Reg – widower at Doctor's Table
Mr Ron Sheehan – gastro; disabled due to car accident

Mrs Royston – colitis; suspected gastro

Mrs Ruby Wilson – high blood pressure. Husband, Neil, alcoholic

Steve – bearded lefty. Wife, Jude

Mr Wayfield – persistent cough

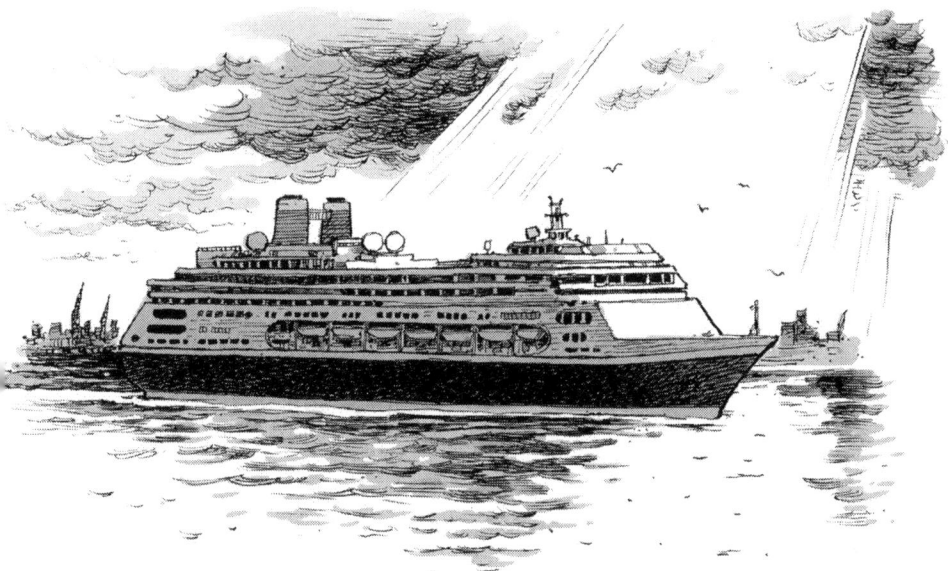

Day 1

Mrs Plummer

'The first experience can never be repeated. The first love, the first sunrise, the first South Sea Island, are memories apart and touch a virginity of sense. (An) interval was passed on deck in the silence of expectation...'

In the South Seas, Robert Louis Stevenson.

I push open the door and step inside a two-bedded ward to find a body lying under a crumpled sheet, pale arm dangling.

Is there rise and fall of the chest? I hold my breath and hurry over, mentally rehearsing my A, B, C, D:

Airway, Breathing, Circulation, D. What the heck does 'D' stand for?

My expensive Advanced Life Support Certificate doesn't stop my heart pounding as I prepare to raise the alarm and bark instructions at a team of resuscitators.

1

Then I realise it's a manikin: a waxen model used for resuscitation training. I breathe out, turn, and shut the door behind me.

⚓

'The dead bodies must have been disembarked,' I tell Tom, my husband. 'The last doctor's gone. Now I can't find out why he let his passengers die. Fancy the receptionist telling us they were waiting for the undertakers.'

Tom is unpacking, hanging suits in the wardrobe. He loves Armani suits. Very dapper. Like Dad. It makes me wonder if all daughters marry some replica of their fathers.

'The nurses will know what happened to the dead passengers. Ask them. Anyway, the bathroom's good – have you seen? Look. We've got a *real* bath.' The bath excites Tom. He can sit in hot water reading for an hour while *The Guardian* becomes sodden.

Our large carpeted cabin, painted in suburban magnolia, boasts a proper double bed, an admirably distressed brown leather sofa, a tiny fridge, and three big portholes with a view of the dock. I try each porthole. They don't budge.

'Oh no,' I grunt. 'No fresh air. I used to love sticking my head out of the portholes.'

It was a different matter on the five crossings our family made to and from Australia in the 1940s, '50s and '60s. Don't ask me how, but Dad managed to wangle the trips as Ten Pound Poms *twice*. He did things like that. Maybe it was because he was a 'super-salesman' who could talk his way into or out of any situation. The family folklore asserted that he could sell sand to Arabs in the desert.

One of my favourite cabin games was to open wide the portholes to feel the needles of sea spray on my face and hear the roar of the engines. Now the big brass wing nuts were screwed down hard onto fat bolts. No shifting them. Here, on the lowest passenger deck, just above the waterline, the opening of portholes was presumably forbidden on Health and Safety grounds, as well as to avoid interference with the cabin's air-conditioning. I don't imagine there was any air-con in the cabins on Harland and Wolff's S.S. *Asturias* in 1949, but there was plenty of fresh air from the portholes when the sea wasn't too rough to splash in. In port my parents would lean out to their waists to talk to friends on the quay.

We are off to Rio. A working holiday for me; a delicious twenty-day break, part of sabbatical leave after fifteen years of twelve-hour days as a GP in Newham.

Poor old Newham, a needy and underfunded east London borough: its people a mix of black and white working class, immigrants and those unfortunates who'd fallen down the social scale and through the moth-eaten welfare net until they'd sunk to the bottom. At least here my patients will be wealthy and therefore healthy, and happy, and I can put my feet up at last. I can't wait to show off my new red bathing costume and stretch myself out on a lounger by the pool, in between reassuring the worried well in surgery. What an excellent idea this is!

~ ⚓ ~

Dr Wallis, the company's Medical Director, is a compact man with a trim moustache and an upright military bearing. 'Splendid, splendid,' was his habitual response to my replies to his interview questions.

He recruited me over the phone, saying I was 'just the sort of doctor' they wanted. I wondered whether my appointment was more related to the fact that I owned my own canal boat on the River Great Ouse. In fact, Dr Wallis seemed to think that with such experience, I was qualified to take over from the captain in an emergency.

When he'd shown us over the ship the previous month, he'd treated Tom and me to an all-you-can-eat buffet in the Officers' Mess. Just in time for lunch, this is where Tom and I are now seated, high up on one of the top decks. The Mess looks out over Southampton's overcast January quayside.

Next to the ship we can see the warehouse where we checked in, a massive cold space big enough to house a jumbo jet. I think about the security officer grinning at me as she'd tucked a stray lock of hair behind her ear: 'You must be the comedienne.'

'No. Doctor,' I'd said.

Looking down, she'd frowned then run her eyes and index finger down the manifest on the trestle table. Tom and I had exchanged glances.

'Ah. Here you are,' she'd said, looking pleased with herself. She'd turned to Tom. 'And you're the doctor?'

'No. My wife is the doctor,' Tom had said.

Passing her finger down the list, the officer finally located Tom's entry with a click of her tongue and a shake of her head, and crossed his name off the manifest as A. N. Other.

Suddenly out of the Mess windows, the clouds part, allowing an ethereal ray of sunshine to dart along the sea road. I interpret it as an omen that all will be well.

The Mess seats thirty people and is open to Senior and Junior Officers at all times of the day and night. Meals are served by specially appointed stewards in neatly pressed white trousers and short jackets. Morning coffee and afternoon tea are laid on with wicked waist-expanding cakes and buns. A yellow sofa and armchair, a coffee table and a television occupy a neat sitting room at one end. Doors lead from there on one side into the Bridge and on the opposite side out to the deck. Extending out from the deck is a curious wing of the ship that forms a viewing platform, which allows the captain or navigation officer to observe the whole length of the ship when the pilot vessel is drawing alongside, or during the hazardous manoeuvre of mooring.

The atmosphere conjures up the long-forgotten smell of a ship's dining room: warm bread rolls and soup.

I heap a luxurious quantity of smoked salmon and salad onto my dinner plate. *Smoked salmon. I mean.* Every day? A bit different to the peanut butter and tomato sandwiches eaten over lunchtime paperwork for the previous fifteen years.

Along the corridor a few steps from our cabin, I open the door to the Medical Centre. Nurse Coralie is at the desk. I ask about the bodies. 'Oh. Them,' she says. 'One was a heart attack, the other – don't know. Coroner's case. Happened three days in – the two of them. Anyhow,' she says, looking at me from under her fringe, 'have you got your uniform?'

'No. Should I have?' Was I supposed to have bought a uniform? From a marine outfitters? I imagine myself in an admiral's outfit with oodles of gold braid and a tricorn hat. Hats suit me.

'It's OK,' Nurse Coralie says. 'Dayap'll fix you up. He's the tailor.'

She gives me rapid-fire directions to the tailor's office, making right and left gestures like semaphore.

A feeling of mild panic sets in.

I'd made up a clever mnemonic to differentiate port from starboard, but now I can't bring it to mind. Was the right-hand side of the ship port because it has an 'r' and a 't' in it, or was the right-side starboard because it possesses two 'r's?

Out in the lobby I prise open a heavy metal door marked 'Crew Only', which leads down metal stairs. Straining to recall Coralie's directions, I trudge along a series of identical grey corridors dully lit by long fluorescent ceiling lights. A crewman with a china-doll face and jet-black hair walks towards me. 'Excuse me. Do you know where I can find the tailor?'

'Tai'or? Yes ma'am. Follow me.' *Ma'am*, he'd said. Now we are getting somewhere. I freely admit that after years of working in the East End of London I am enjoying my new elevated status. If I'd have been called madam in Newham, it would have meant something entirely different.

Following china-doll man past crew cabins with poster-sized 'DO NOT DISTURB' signs on the doors, along more corridors and down another grey metal staircase, I wonder how I'm ever going to find my way back alone.

Aged two and three-quarters, on our first sea voyage, I had adoringly followed our motherly Italian cabin stewardess, Maria, who pinched my fat cheeks and pronounced me *bella*. One day tailing her on her rounds I was deemed missing. Panic. There were announcements over the tannoy and frantic searches along corridors and in storerooms. Passengers looked over the side. When Mum found me in a cabin with Maria she cried and hugged me so tight that I could hardly breathe.

Dayap's workshop shares the same below-the-waterline space as the ship's laundry: a football-pitch-sized windowless steam factory of linen, towels, and uniforms in all stages of washing and ironing. Ten male launderers, sweating in once-white vests and trousers, operate huge roller irons amid the industrial, glue-sniffing smell of dry-cleaning machines.

'Hello. I've come for my uniform… doctor.'

Dayap, with a sun-beaten, brown face, no trace of a beard, and thick, straight, black hair, his hairline as low as an eight-year-old boy's, sits in the small workshop that doubles as a uniform store. On his sewing table, with its photograph of a woman and three children, coloured threads, buttons, and braid, he appears to be on guard against any intruder who might attempt to help themselves to his stock. Hung up on packed rails and sitting on the floor in cardboard boxes lay the ready-to-wear outfits for hundreds of crew.

'Dottor?' He raises his eyes.

'Yes. *Doctor.*'

'Size?' He breathes out loudly through his nose.

'Usually I'm a twelve, but it depends on the make and cut.'

Dayap looks unimpressed. Clearly the last thing he wants is to interrupt machining a massive green velvet curtain, but he rises slowly and looks me up and down, down and up.

'Try this.' He thrusts a dark blue skirt into my hands.

I look round for a place to change but realise I am in it.

Behind a rack of tropically coloured, multi-layered skirts I discover that the tight blue skirt sits well above my knees. Not only do I have Dad's knobbly knees, but I definitely don't want the public to see my Hoxton market knickers as I bend over a fallen passenger. Maybe I should buy myself some glamorous knickers from the ship's boutique. No. There is nothing for it but to ask for the skirt's hem to be let down. Dayap avoids my gaze then passes me a somewhat ill-fitting pair of men's serge trousers as an alternative, while promising to attend to the skirt's hem the next day.

'Here.'

He hands me a heavy navy jacket with gold and red striped braid on the sleeves. It fits. I pull on an enormous white shirt, then one that's too tight to button up. Clicking his tongue, he picks out three work shirts, a long black skirt, a fancy formal shirt, and a cream bolero jacket, advising himself aloud on which ones to choose in his own language, which sounds like Spanish with too many 'a's and glottal stops. Muttering, he signs out the stock in a big red record book lying on a specially designed shelf just inside the door, with its biro hanging on a string. He packs me off dressed in what passes for the male doctor's day uniform, with spare shirts, my other clothes and the formal evening outfit balanced across my arms.

Hurrying back through the passenger area, I bump into a man who steps out of his cabin with his wife close behind, beaming.

'Are you in charge of the chambermaids?' he asks.

'No. I'm the doctor.' I pull myself up to my full height and puff out my chest, hoping that he notices my DOCTOR name badge.

'Well, I just wanted to let you know that they've done a *marvellous* job, really *marvellous* – we've just been moved!' He grins broadly, his face crinkling. 'Thank you.'

'Oh good,' I mutter. At least he assumes I am in charge of *something*.

'Is *that* your uniform?' Tom asks, clearly unimpressed. I recount the tale of the too-short-skirt and the chambermaid incident.

Reaching up, I open a top cupboard, grab my lucky blue stethoscope and quickly turn to go. Thwack! Tom yelps. He is bending forward, nursing his forehead and groaning.

'Couldn't you see the door was open?' I rail. 'Look what you're doing! You never look!'

'Oh, I see. So, it's *my* fault!'

We glare at each other.

Here I am on this death ship, mistaken for a comedienne,

then a chambermaid, dressed as a man, and accompanied by an accident-prone husband who would very likely show me up by falling overboard.

Whose idea was this whole cruise ship thing anyway?

I march round to the Medical Centre, sit down hard on the consulting room chair and glower at the corkboard. Twenty days to go.

—⚓—

Tilbury, 1952

We left port with the ship growling and starting to roll.

I, alongside hundreds of other passengers, held tightly to the end of a coloured streamer, having thrown the other end to my uncle and aunt on the quay. As the ship started to move, the streamers were gradually pulled apart between our two hands, Uncle Harry waving his torn end until he became a dot on the dockside. No coloured streamers breaking in the hands of loved ones on the shore now. No waving of white hankies until no longer distinguishable in the haze. We were heading back to Australia to take up our lives once more, Mum unaware that she would see her brother Harry, her other four brothers and sister again, but never her mother.

—⚓—

Stiff-backed, shoulders hunched, I await my first patient. I am determined that no-one is going to die on my watch.

First through the door is Mrs Plummer, a tall, distinguished-looking woman in her fifties with immaculate eye makeup and red glossy lipstick. She wears a royal blue power dress, and smells of coconut.

'I've had some tests with my GP and he phoned me with the results yesterday, but I didn't have time to collect the medication. I wondered if you'd have it on board? You can ring my doctor and check if you like. I have his number here,' she says, reaching into the black patent handbag on her knees. Then she announces the diagnosis.

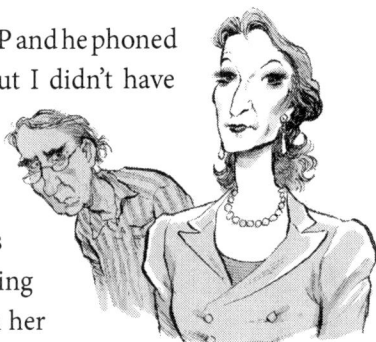

She has caught an exceptionally rare venereal disease, which I had only read about in the small print of a medical textbook as a student, twenty years previously. I have not the slightest idea what to prescribe. I'm nodding, at the same time as stopping my chair from sliding backwards and forwards on its castors in time with the roll of the ship.

'It was just an unfortunate encounter,' she says. 'I've had it before, you know, but, you see, I'm away such a lot with my work. Human resources. My husband knows. He's *very* understanding.' She moistens her lips.

'I'm sure we can help,' I hear myself say, relying heavily on the royal plural.

As my chair approaches the shelf above the desk I reach for the medication bible – the British National Formulary and open it. With a rush of relief, I find the exact diagnosis listed in the index, and the drugs spelled out in detail on the page.

Nurse Coralie checks our tiny pharmacy. Good news. The medication is in stock. *Tablets or injections, Mrs Plummer? Tablets.* It is going to be a long course. Coralie dispenses 144 bitter pills. This is not the NHS. Coralie adds £128.50 to Mrs Plummer's account. Mrs Plummer doesn't blink.

'*So* well stocked. Mr Plummer *will* be relieved,' she says as she stands up.

Mr Wayfield is next.

'I put all my pills on the sideboard ready to go into the case, then I left without them. We were in such a rush, you see, cos the taxi'd arrived.' Mr Wayfield looks flustered, his face blotchy and his buff-coloured travel clothes already crushed.

We rake over the details of his regular medications, those that he can remember – the pill for his blood pressure, which sounds like Anatol, the capsule for his cholesterol, which he thinks is green, the aspirin (that's the easy one), the 'dieseljesus' for his back pain and the blue and brown inhalers. Coralie quickly locates them, dispenses the lot and makes up the bill.

'You've *charged* me to see the doctor. I only *wanted* my prescription. I didn't *need* to see a doctor. Why've I been charged for that?' Mr Wayfield's small eyes glare.

'Well, I have to work out what your drugs are, so as not to prescribe something different and possibly dangerous, and legally I'm responsible for the prescribing.'

'That's not fair. The nurse could have worked it all out from what I told her.'

'The nurse can't prescribe. If she'd got it wrong, I'd have been liable. That's why the fee has to come under a doctor's consultation.'

He leaves with a 'humph', jogging the desk as he gets up.

It's a relief not to be involved in the billing. I am not used to having a monetary relationship with my patients. It doesn't feel right; gets in the way of trust and transparency. A conflict of interest.

The clinic has finished and Coralie bangs the Medical Centre door shut with obvious relief.

'You coming?' She tosses her head to move the fringe out of her eyes.

'Thanks. I'll go to the passengers' dining room with Tom.'

'I'm on tonight so I'll be takin' the calls. I'll let you know if I need you.' She puts away the stapler and pens in the desk, closing the drawer with a sharp clack.

'Okay.'

'Liz'll be on in the morning.'

'Very good.'

It seems like there are other things to be said. Something is missing but I can't tell what. It makes me feel uneasy.

No doctor in her right mind would choose to go on holiday with all her patients. Yet this evening when Mrs Plummer enters the dining-room I learn something that couldn't have been revealed in our consultation. Mr Plummer, trailing Mrs P, tall, stooped, wearing half-moon glasses, looks resigned, or resentful, or is it angry? I don't see them speak to each other at their table for two throughout the whole meal, as they stare across the dining room in opposite directions.

Passengers can ask to be seated at the Doctor's Table when they book their cruise, and that is where they will be installed for the whole twenty-one days. The round table accommodates eight people and commands a view of the rest of the dining room, while the rest of the dining room commands a view of the Doctor's Table. Regulations state that I have to wear uniform in the company of passengers, whereas civvies are acceptable in the Officers' Mess. But in civvies, I am expected to keep out of the public eye and stick to the hopelessly labyrinthine crew corridors, with their lines of identical grey cabin doors and massive storerooms.

Tom, having been mistaken for the doctor three times since embarkation, is relegated to anonymity once we are in public together.

'Oh, so you're the doctor's husband,' they say, losing interest.

Sitting next to me is Reginald. A veteran cruiser, widowed, he is travelling alone. He looks to be in his eighties, with a narrow face, a head of thinning grey hair, the top strands carefully combed forward to his forehead, and a reedy voice. In his dark blue blazer with shiny gold buttons, he smells of cigarettes, which turns my stomach.

'I always book the Doctor's Table,' Reginald says, breathing on me.

'Oh, why's that?' I think of the appeal of my gripping medical anecdotes, and the reflected kudos of my elevated rank.

'Free wine.' He makes an involuntary grunting noise in the back of his throat. 'Ah, but you're new, aren't you? On Formal Nights there's company wine on all the officers' tables. Not tonight. Formal Night's tomorrow.' I don't know whether to think him clever or conniving.

Tom leans over towards Reginald: 'Sounds like you're from Essex. Am I right?'

'Colchester.'

'I know Colchester. I used to have union members in the army barracks there.'

'Get away! In the Garrison?' says Reg. 'I own a storage place near there. D'you know Garrison Road? I'm at the back. We keep a mountain of soldiers' stuff when they move in and when they get posted overseas. It's a blooming good earner, I can tell you. M.O.D. pays. D'you know the Garrison's been there since Roman times. They've still got the Parachute Regiment.'

'Yes, yes, I know,' says Tom. 'One of my members' sons was in the Paras. Once I saw him land on the parade ground during practice.'

'That's the same ground they used in the Monty Python film *Meaning of Life*. Which union is it?'

'Well, I'm retired now but I was an officer in the Engineering and Electrical Union. Staff section. Not that I've ever been an engineer or an electrician, if that makes sense.'

Reginald is losing interest and looks across to a table of women who are laughing loudly.

Tom empties half of his wine glass.

'Where are you from?' he asks the neighbouring couple.

Pam and Derek are both big, very big. They only just squeeze into the green leatherette armchairs, and resemble each other the way couples do when they have the same body type. They are wearing matching nautical tops.

'Us? We're from Portsmouth,' says Derek. 'The ferries – security – port security.'

'I know Portsmouth,' says Tom. 'I used to visit the naval dockyards. They're absolutely *massive. Huge* complex. Enormously high walls; all those eighteenth-century buildings and museum ships...'

'Before then. I mean, they've got the *Mary Rose* there. She's *hundreds* of years old,' says Derek.

'Yes. The *Mary Rose* is fifteen-hundreds,' Pam says, 'easily. She was made from six hundred oak trees – forty acres' worth. I remember that because Buckingham Palace is forty acres. There were two hundred skeletons found in her too, when they brought her up. Poor souls.'

Tom and Derek compare road routes from Portsmouth to Southampton and the surrounding towns like the beginning of an Ayckbourn play. It's a man thing.

Pam wants to talk about her daughters. 'Beth's a teacher. Carol, well, she's taken a while to settle down, hasn't she, Derek? She lives in a squat with musicians, but it's alright. They share everything, even their toothbrushes! ... I know! Carol's very musical. Wonderful voice.'

I visualise the obstetric risks due to Pam's morbid obesity and see myself struggling with her delivery, reverting to an emergency caesarean section in the nick of time, mining the layers as I proceed. Then there is the unmistakeable 'Waaa! Waaa!' That would have been Carol.

An elderly Scots couple sit on the other side of Reg; Jim and

Mary. Mary is quietly spoken with a Highlands accent. She has a round doughnut-shaped face topped by an old-fashioned back-combed hairdo, and wears what looks like an elderly relative's costume jewellery, purple over a pink twinset. She seems rather serious. Jim doesn't say much.

'This is our first cruise,' Mary says. 'Are ye the *doctor* then?' she asks, slightly awed, I think.

'Yes.'

'Well, ye ken, I was in the hospital last year. They were to take out my gallbladder by keyhole, they were, but in theatre they just couldn't fetch it out, so they had to do the cut instead. I was *so ill* afterwards. They made me stay for *two weeks*. The surgeon said he'd never *seen* so many stones. But Carol managed to sell them on eBay – for jewellery – which was nice.'

I 'mmed' the way doctors are trained to do.

Jim looks at Mary, chiding. 'Och, doctor doesn't want to talk shop at the dinner table, Mary.'

'I'm sure she doesn't mind,' says Mary, looking at me, 'do ye?'

Food starts to arrive. The smell of oxtail soup brings me to my feet. The sea is heaving. Waves of nausea wash into the back of my throat.

'Excuse me. I need to get hold of the nurse to sort out something... sorry...'

I'd suffered from motion sickness for as long as I could remember. Many a car seat and carpet had been spoiled. Mum resorted to making me suck barley sugar at the start of a journey. She must have heard about it as a home remedy on the wireless. But the barley sugar just came back and, Pavlov-like, even the smell of barley sugar became firmly associated in my nostrils with the need to vomit. A hundred yards in the back of a car could set me off. However, I'd also inherited Dad's wanderlust: a restless man always wanting variety and adventure. So did I, enough to put up with a little travel sickness. It was a temporary thing. Even Charles Darwin, during his five-year voyage on H.M.S. *Beagle,* suffered from sea-sickness at a time when there were no effective remedies. '*I was resolved to go at all hazards,*' Darwin records in his diary. '*I had no doubt I should frequently repent of the whole undertaking, little did I think with what fervour I should do so.*' And, just as he had anticipated, many '*days were ones of great & unceasing suffering*'. But look where his journeys took him.

—⚓—

Thirty minutes later, Tom comes into the cabin. 'Oh darling. You look awful!'

'Thanks. Just let me be,' I moan, lying on top of the bed in my uniform. 'I just want to sleep.'

'What about some tea?' Tom sits on the edge of the bed and takes my hand.

'Urrgh. No thanks.'

'Water?'

'*No-o.*'

'You have to try *something.*'

'I've tried *loads* of things before. Nothing *works.*' Even talking makes me feel like throwing up. I want the ship to be clear of the bucking Bay of Biscay.

Tom disappears and comes back five minutes later with a small packet.

'Come on now. Sit up. Take one of these.' He uses his commanding voice.

'What is it?'

'It's a *sea-sick pill.* I got it at reception.'

'What's it called?'

'I don't *know*... S – Stugeron.' Tom reads it out as if it's a foreign language.

'Never heard of it. Is that the proper name?'

'Don't ask *me*! *You* have a look. Here's the packet.'

I focus. 'Cinn-ar-izine. Never heard of it.'

'Just *try* it,' he says, his voice a falsetto of frustration.

'If it comes back up, don't say I didn't warn you.'

Sitting up, I swallow the tiny pill with a sip of water, then slump down, sighing like a punctured lifejacket.

After dinner Tom is standing by the bed. I open one eye.

'How are you feeling?'

'Let me see.' I prop myself up onto one elbow. 'Mm. Better... I think.'

'You see. You're *so* stubborn.'

'Well. Nothing's ever worked before.'

I feel somehow resentful that after all my years of suffering he has so readily found a pill that actually works.

―⚓―

Southampton, 1969

I thought myself tremendously lucky to get a job as a nurse (my first qualifications) on one of the biggest one-class passenger ships in the world. With just three days' notice I was recruited over the phone. Once on board, it became abundantly clear why the company had not waited to check my nursing credentials nor obtained references. The organisation was chaotic. Crossing the Bay of Biscay, I lay on the hospital operating table, grey-green with nausea, until the ship tossed me onto the linoleum. After that I lay on the floor. When the hospital bell rang, I'd struggle to my feet, trying not to throw up, to treat passengers for sea-sickness. I wanted to die. I really wouldn't have minded.

But when the feeling had passed, I was glad I hadn't. I got to sail around the world, like Charles Darwin.

⚓

Up on deck the cool, clean breeze brushes my face. Clouds scud across the bright full moon. It looks like the silver fragments have fallen into the black sea, where they bob and glimmer on the waves. It makes me think of Dad.

He was fifteen before he first saw the sea. He'd cycled to Southend with his best friend, Les. The sea looked gun-metal grey under an overcast sky but the immensity and mystery of it brought him and Les back again and again. The more he saw of the sea, the more Dad became enamoured with it. He dreamed of living near water. After we returned to England from Australia in 1956, Dad would organise boating holidays on the Broads, the Thames and the Dutch canals. His love of waterways and boats seeped into my blood.

⚓

The evening show has just started in the Ocean Lounge, a small amphitheatre with banked tiers of plush red velvet seats served by small tables, divided by large pillars and overlooked by sparkling chandeliers.

On stage is a diminutive, bubbly brunette in her forties, calling herself Magic Moll. She has a high-pitched voice, one that you payed attention to, theatrically projected. The comedienne. Nothing like me at all. She calls for a volunteer.

'Ooh, look at you, half man, half deckchair,' she trills as Mr Plummer climbs up on stage in a blue and white striped shirt. 'And what do we call you, sir?' She leans into his personal space.

'Arthur.' He has a deep voice and being about six feet tall, he bends his head towards her.

'Arthur. That's nice – Arthur. I see you've got a lovely watch, Arthur. Might I borrow it?'

Arthur takes his watch off and hands it to Moll.

Moll puts it in a cloth, steps back to a small table and bashes it to smithereens with a mallet. There is a pause for gasps and laughter. Then, after a spell, she walks up to Arthur at the front of the stage and says, 'Ooh, Arthur, you know what, Arthur?... Eh, guess what?... I can't *remember* the rest of the trick.' She sucks her breath in through pursed lips, eyes wide, and pauses for effect. 'Ooh, your *watch*, Arthur. What *are* we gonna do?'

Arthur blinks, looking anxious and perplexed.

'Is that your wife in the next seat, Arthur?' Moll points.

Arthur looks over as if to be sure. 'Yes, that's her.'

'Tell you what, Arthur, we'd better find a replacement watch quick smart, or your wife will be *wild*. What do you say?' She looks up at him with a grave face.

Arthur mutters, 'Yes, I think so.' Upon which, with a dramatic movement, Moll reaches over and produces the watch, apparently unharmed, from Arthur's shirt pocket.

Arthur smiles and lets out a sigh. Moll unexpectedly kisses his cheek and the audience applaud loudly.

Time to explore the next deck up. In the bar we find a woman singer accompanied by a guitarist in full swing. Better still, there's a little dancefloor surrounded by tables and chairs. Dark wood panelling covers the lower half of three walls, on the upper part of which modern paintings are displayed. A long, curved bar with polished brass fittings, a mirror-shine-top and two bartenders occupies the remaining side. The singer has a voice as clear and crisp as a glass bell and the guitarist is an expert. As dedicated dancers we've struck gold. Nothing is going to stop us from getting on the floor, uniform or no uniform.

Tom had been the jumping-jack-jiver with the twinkly eyes in a sweat-stained t-shirt at the 100 Club in London's Oxford Street. It's still there. If he hadn't twinkled at me that night, none of this would have happened. I had been one of those little girls sent to ballet lessons at the age of six, and by the time I was thirteen I was attending ballroom dancing classes. Going out dancing was the way to meet boys. From Dennis Drew's Dance Academy in Upton Park, east London, in the 1980s, I felt right up to speed with jive, boasting the blue ribbon prize in the silver medal exam. Tom and I both loved to show off and had developed a complementary dance style that suited our showmanship.

The duo sound like *The Carpenters*, the 1960s' brother and sister duo, and are singing *Top of the World*, the woman slapping a tambourine rhythmically against her thigh. As we jive, the duo play *Please Mr Postman* for us. Grasping each other's hands, we swing out and back, round and round, then close hold, delighted to be snugly up against each other for those few seconds, we swing out again, exchanging snatches of conversation. 'What do you think?' Tom asks.

'Oh, just wonderful,' I say, 'and the singer is *really* good. A bit Joni Mitchell.'

I like the way the duo introduces their songs, rather than just starting a number without giving any information about the original singer or the song. Next comes The Beatles' *Ticket to Ride*, and we give it everything we have left from the day. The duo smile and nod. As I whirl off Tom's arm, this whole cruise idea suddenly seems exceptionally fine.

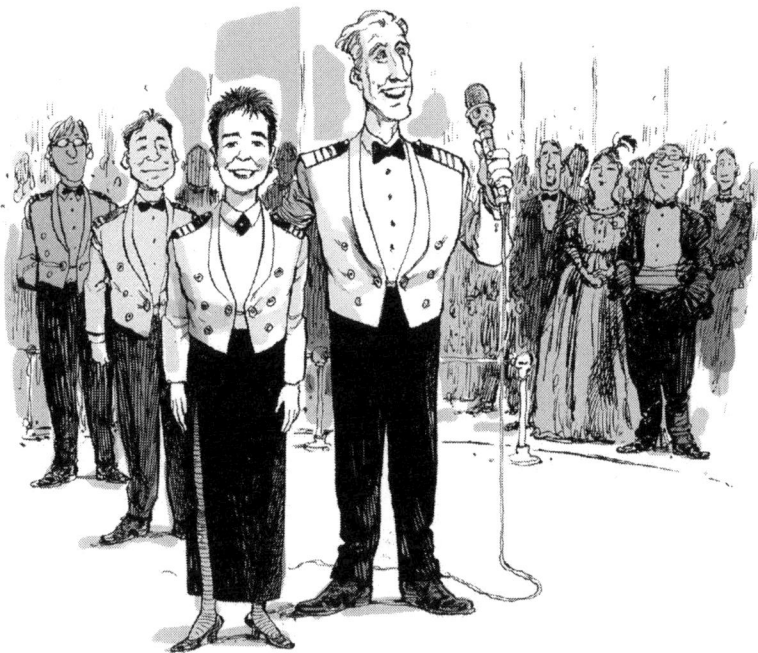

Day 2

Mr Wayfield

The Bay of Biscay, stretching from Brittany to northern Spain, is shaped like Don Quixote's shaving bowl. The exposed western side attracts wind and waves from the Atlantic, which become trapped, swirling in a dizzy race around the basin. The edges are formed from the continental shelves of France and Spain, while the centre plunges to a bone-crushing five thousand metres, beyond the reach of most sea creatures. Above, warm air carried by the Gulf Stream meets cold water, creating high winds. *Sea Rainbow* has to cross this whirlpool. Fortunately, she is fitted with stabilisers. Metal fins below the water line alter their angles to counteract the roll. The first major cruise liner to be fitted with stabilisers was the 48,000-ton luxury Italian S.S. *Conte di Savoia* in 1932. I discover that *Sea Rainbow*'s 35,000-ton motion can't be entirely controlled by its modern stabilisers seventy years later.

Collecting grapefruit juice from the cool unit in the dining room, I notice an uncorked bottle of champagne sitting in an ice bucket with flutes beside it. A passenger makes herself a Buck's fizz and another splashes champagne into his half-filled glass until it bubbles over.

What! Alcohol for breakfast?

Alcoholism statistics and years of anti-alcohol health education ricochet round my brain. Surely it's my duty to warn the passengers of the dangers, such as the fifty percent rise in alcoholic liver cirrhosis and alcohol-related early deaths in Britain, the increasing annual costs to the NHS, or at least remind people of their weekly limit in units? Not at seven-thirty in the morning. I cross to the bran flakes dispenser.

Apparently, there is always champagne for breakfast on a Formal Night. It is definitely not for me at this time of the morning. I'd nod off in the middle of the first consultation, or before it. Wouldn't look good.

Liz is in the Medical Centre arranging files on the desk when I arrive. Slim, dark-haired and in her late thirties, her first words are, 'Hi Doc. Listen, we've had a couple of gastros in the night... Coralie saw them and gave them all the stuff.'

'What stuff?'

'You know – the form to fill out, Lomotil, anti-emetics, stool pot... Oh, this is your first cruise, isn't it? It's all in the Protocol Book. Here...' She hands me a heavy green lever-arch file marked 'PROTOCOLS'.

'We put the names in the gastro log over there.' Liz points to the filing cabinet. 'We'll ring people tonight and see how they're doing. I *really* hope they're our only ones.'

She looks concerned in a way that I don't follow. Gastroenteritis is one of the commonest minor illnesses in General Practice. So what?

The phone starts to ring.

'When did it start?... How many times?... Stay in your cabin... No, *don't* come down to the Medical Centre. Doctor will come up to you,' I hear Liz repeat with each call.

Three more cases are logged.

Coralie arrives and immediately leaves to do water testing. The water in the pools and jacuzzis is tested daily for noxious microbes.

'Here are your gastros,' Coralie announces on her return, handing me a bunch of notes she's gathered from the office. She smells of cigarettes and her broad face has that lived-in look that smokers get, with little lines around the eyes and tiny blood vessels visible under the skin of her cheeks.

Coralie and Liz are busy checking the controlled drugs. The drugs safe is wide open while Liz records the results, balancing the over-large drugs book on her knees. I grab gloves, plastic aprons and the gastro equipment bag. I need to visit the patients to confirm the diagnosis and to make sure passengers are not so ill that they require admission to our miniature hospital.

It takes me over an hour to find the cabins, don fresh gloves and plastic apron for each patient, see all three passengers and their travelling companions, elicit the patients' histories, and give them and their companions instructions about managing gastroenteritis. They are sentenced to isolation. When passengers see that the doctor is visiting, their accounts can be long-winded, to which they add their friends' or family members' traumatic or wonderful NHS experiences. By now I'm hungry and irritable.

I want to be with Tom, enjoying smoked salmon salad, exchanging experiences of the morning and laughing. I badly want to laugh.

When I get back to the Medical Centre, there is a message on the desk. Coralie and Liz have gone to lunch.

Something about the nurses' behaviour makes me feel uneasy. Why aren't we the happy close-knit cooperative team I'd expected? They're not exactly hostile. Maybe it is just me. My tendency to be reserved until I get to know people can come across as haughty.

The ship, still in the Bay of Biscay, is rocking up and down like a lift that keeps missing its floor. It makes my stomach lurch.

***

In the afternoon Liz, Coralie and I ring all the gastros. One passenger is keen for release. She has suffered from an intestinal complaint for years and asserts that this is the cause of her stomach upset. She feels fine. According to the lever-arch file, she is to stay put until the following morning to be sure her symptoms subside. Liz puts her hand over the telephone mouthpiece. 'Would you speak to her?'

'Can't I at least go to the Captain's Cocktail Party tonight?' she protests. 'I promise I'll come straight back to the cabin afterwards.' Firm, but wheedling.

'Sorry, you can't. We have to be sure that you are completely better before releasing you,' I say, trying to sound like Dr Evidence-Based-Care.

'But that's *ridiculous*. I've had Crohn's disease for years. I was only reporting it in case it got out of hand and you had to give me more tablets. I shouldn't be penalised for doing the right thing,' she continues in a plaintive tone.

'It's ship's policy. You understand that if you develop more symptoms overnight you *could* be infectious,' says Dr Official-Protocol.

'I'm telling you *there's no way* that I'm infectious. Can't you just *ask* if my husband and I can at *least* have champagne and canapés in the cabin. We'll be missing the best meal of the week as it is. Room-service food is just *awful*.'

I'm getting nowhere.

'OK. I'll ask the Hotel Manager to contact you. You can discuss it with him,' says Dr Passing-the-Buck.

I know exactly what the answer will be.

I bleep Oleg.

'You are joking.'

'I've told her it's not possible, ship's policy and all that, but she won't take no for an answer. Would you mind speaking to her? She needs the Word of God.'

I know he won't be able to resist being elevated to such heights of authority.

~⚓~

At evening surgery Mr Wayfield is back with an irritating cough. Every time he coughs his bald head grows redder and shinier. He is in the same crushed beige travel clothes as yesterday.

On examination there are no signs of a chest infection or exacerbation of his asthma, but he stresses that he is embarrassed by the cough at the dinner table. I prescribe a cough mixture, more as a placebo than anything else, and give him advice about sucking hard sweets and moisturising the dry cabin air.

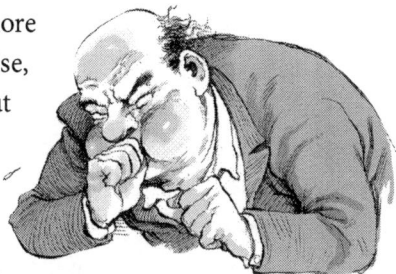

Coralie appears at the

consulting room door to tell me that I must be in my formal uniform in half an hour to be presented to the passengers by the Master at the Captain's Welcome Cocktail Party. I've already missed the first sitting.

'You might have told me, Coralie. Don't let me miss things I'm supposed to attend.'

'You'll've had an e-mail about it. Didn't you look at yer e-mails?' Coralie is unblinking.

'Well, where do I find the e-mails?'

She shows me. There the e-mail sits, staring at me from the Hotel Manager.

***

I burst into our cabin. 'Guess what? I was supposed to be at first sitting Captain's Cocktail Party and nobody said. Now I'll have to rush like mad to get to second sitting. I've got to be presented to the passengers. How embarrassing. *Really.*'

'Can I do anything?' Tom asks, as he comes up to kiss me.

'No thanks, I'll just get moving,' I say, bestowing a passing peck.

Tom opens the wardrobe and is looking at his dinner suit, bow tie in hand. 'D'you know what *I've* done?'

'What *now*?' I stop, one leg in, one leg out of my skirt.

'No dinner jacket.' He lifts up the hanger that holds his dress trousers to show me.

'*What?*'

'I haven't packed my dinner jacket. That's *what.*'

'For goodness' sake! Go up to the boutique and see if they've got one.'

'They won't have my size. Nobody *ever* has my size. It'll be a complete waste of time.'

'Well, just *go* and *have a look*. Do you want me to come with you?' I start putting my leg back into the skirt.

'No. *I'll* go. You're late. Get ready.' He throws the hanger on the bed and dashes off, letting the door slam.

Once the uniform black evening skirt is zipped up, I notice it has a long sexy slit up one side to my thigh; right up to my stocking tops. What on earth...? Patients are supposed to undress for the doctor, not the other way round. Aplomb. That's all I can employ in this situation. Dressed in the slit skirt, white pleated dress shirt with cuff links, black bow tie, double-breasted cream bolero jacket with brass buttons and red and gold epaulettes, stockings and black high-heeled shoes, I trip along to the Ocean Lounge, holding my head high. Why the heck haven't I brought tights? Oh yes – because we're going to Rio. Clasping the edges of the skirt's slit firmly together with one hand, I slide past lines of glamorously clad passengers queuing outside the lounge, waiting to be allowed in.

There is a buzz of excitement amid the heavy scent of perfume as they press up against each other, chattering and chuckling, the women in long evening gowns – one is a gorgeous silky, blue, backless number, reminiscent of the 1930s, clingy, with a flare of material as it flows to the floor. I imagine myself, with a different body and a replacement head, doing an elegant slow foxtrot, taking those long gliding strides backwards, head up and to the left, back arched. How I'd avoid tripping on the train doesn't concern me. The men are wearing black dinner suits – much less inspiring, except for some flamboyant extroverts who sport cherry-spotted bow ties.

The captain, with his tell-tale four-striped epaulettes, is standing with some of the officers inside the lounge. As the captain's eye catches mine, I say, 'Sorry I missed first sitting – saving lives you know,' and smile in contrition.

'Oh, I see,' he says, looking grave.

The ship is rolling, side to side, side to side.

I swallow half a cinnarizine, which I've slipped into my

jacket pocket, then introduce myself properly to the captain.

'Yes, I knew it was you. Welcome aboard,' beams the warm Norwegian, squeezing my hand with just the right amount of reassuring pressure. He confirms my name, written on a small slip of paper he holds.

The doors to the lounge swing open and the first passengers walk up the slope, shake hands with the captain and have their photos taken with him by the on-board photographer standing in front of a huge backdrop displaying a vivid orange sunset over an ocean. This ritual continues for half an hour. Captain Strom's smile on his angular face looks fresh for every photo. Must have undergone advanced smile training. Probably has the certificate. We officers line up and greet the passengers in turn. Some seasoned cruisers know the Cruise Director and Hotel Manager so well that hearty 'How are *you*?'s and 'Great to *see* you again!'s are exchanged, amid updating gossip and laughter.

The half tablet does not entirely prevent nausea as I find myself attempting to stifle a succession of burps. It does, however, produce its sedative effect, making me yawn uncontrollably. Actually, I'm starting to feel faint. I can sense the blood draining from my face. I take deep breaths while flexing my feet repeatedly to drive the circulation back up to my brain. How I wish I'd been able to get hold of the legendary Coast Guard Cocktail: a mixture of equal parts of promethazine for nausea, which is sedative, and ephedrine, a stimulant known as 'speed'. Just the ticket.

⚓

A woman in a blue sequinned gown and bobbing feather fascinator approaches me. 'It's so *good* to see a woman doctor on board for a change,' she says, smiling. Presumably she recognises the red and gold doctor's epaulettes from previous cruises. Seasoned passengers do.

A short man whose red cummerbund is stretched tightly over his full waist walks up to me with hail-fellow-well-met eagerness.

He shakes my hand. 'Where are you from?'

'London – I'm a GP in east London. It's what's called challenging,' I confide.

'I imagine so. Have you heard of the Royal Society of Apothecaries?'

'No.'

'We're in Blackfriars. You live in London, you say?'

I nod as a gentle burp erupts.

'You know the Society was actually founded in 1617. Absolutely *wonderful*. *Terrific* lectures. You must go. Don't forget. The Royal Society of Apothecaries. Look them up when you get home.'

'I will. How interesting,' I say, suppressing a yawn.

It seems odd to me that he views us as colleagues. But maybe we are. I presume that apothecaries are all pharmacists, or were – and in the City of London, posh pharmacists. In 1617 they would have been the local chemists, fabricating all sorts of curious concoctions such as mixtures to remove moss from gravestones, and potions of herbs and animal parts to treat a spectrum of diseases that were not understood. The forerunners of today's GPs.

Tom appears sporting a delectable cream dinner jacket that fits him perfectly. Any resemblance to James Bond is purely coincidental. We exchange admiring glances.

The captain straightens his jacket. The Cruise Director nods to the orchestra, which strikes up a fanfare. 'And the moment you've all been waiting for. I'd like you to give a very warm welcome to the Master of the Ship – Captain Ivor Strom!'

The Cruise Director throws his arm in the captain's direction.

Captain Strom walks coolly up the aisle between rows of passengers. They look up from their canapés. He has the air of a man in charge, perfectly at ease.

'Good evening, ladies and gentlemen, and a very big welcome to you all. Well, we have a wonderful cruise ahead of us with many exciting ports. Some of you lucky cruisers are all-rounders, and others are staying with us until the end of the first section in Rio. Right now, we have just entered the Bay of Biscay and fortunately we have only light seas and a southwest breeze of fifteen knots. Not too bad. Now, one of the things passengers always ask me is why a ship is called 'she'. Let me tell you. It is because she needs a lick of paint to look her best, when she enters the harbour she always heads for the buoys, and it takes a good man to handle her.'

He pauses for the laughter to die down.

'We have a wonderful crew on board. Always smiling.'

Applause.

'We are a family of fourteen nations.'

More applause.

'I would like to introduce you to every one of them, but I know some of you wouldn't want to miss your dinner.'

Chuckles.

'So tonight, I am going to present the Senior Officers who keep the ship running. First up is our Chief Officer: Tallak Steensen.'

Tallak strides steadily up onto the stage to the audience's applause, his heavy black shoes pinning him to the floor like a moonwalker.

'So where are you from, Tallak?' The captain turns to face him.

'From Sølvefjord in Norway.' It sounds rehearsed. They must have said the same thing at the first sitting.

'Ah, you see, Tallak is my neighbour. We see each other's houses across the fjord. Isn't that so?'

'Yes, we do.'

'Not only that, but Tallak is a fully trained captain himself. His name means 'contender' in Norwegian, so when I'm walking downstairs, I have to be very careful to watch my back.' Captain Strom looks to the audience for sympathy.

'So – if you find *any* problems with the cruise or have any complaints, don't hesitate to tell Tallak about them.'

Further laughter.

The captain glances at the piece of paper in his hand.

'Next up is an officer who hopes not to do any work during the cruise. We have our doctor – Ruth Taylor.'

Polite applause.

I wobble up onto the stage, swaying slightly. So, let them see the stocking tops. I am past caring. I'm aware from the drained feeling in my face that I must look pale, even sickly, with my thick black eyebrows standing out, one surprised, the other supercilious. I stopped plucking them thirty years back when I discovered that it hurt. Why would I want the eyebrows of a seven-year-old anyway?

'And where do you come from?'

'From England – London.'

Loud applause and cheering.

'And how do you like to be called?'

'Errm… Dr Ruth.'

A ripple of titters erupts from those familiar with American television personality Dr Ruth, of sexual therapy fame.

Instantly I regret my response. Do I really want the world turning up to the Medical Centre for advice about their sexual problems? Especially in view of the stocking tops. They'd have been far better off seeing the Cruise Director, Eric West. He looks understanding. Captain Strom, unfazed, introduces the other Senior Officers, who take their places next to him and me, and he finally calls the head chef.

'Lenz Burger – he does cook other things as well… So how many chefs have you in the kitchen?' Captain Strom looks along the line at Lenz, who stands at the end.

'Sixty-four.'

Gasps.

'Sixty-four chefs? How do you keep so many chefs in order?'

'You know, I have fifteen rolling pins, and as well, there are plenty of sharp knives handy.'

Sniggers.

'No,' Lenz continues, 'I can say that we all get on great. We have to when we make four and a half thousand meals a day.'

Women gasp.

'Well, ladies and gentlemen – I think I can hear stomachs rumbling now, and I don't want to keep you from your dinners any longer. So, I wish you all a wonderful cruise. Thank you for your attention.'

***

Pam and Derek are already seated when we get to our table. Derek is in his black dress suit with a radical white bow tie. Pam's silky dress covered in coloured swirls is very low cut. Reginald, Jim and Mary arrive together. Our waiter, Manas, in his well-pressed black trousers and white cropped jacket, pulls out the women's chairs.

'Och, don't *ye* look smart,' Mary says. 'Do ye have to bring your own uniform?'

She puts her black satin evening bag on the table. It matches her dress, which has chiffon sleeves. John's suit looks like his Sunday best – dark blue accompanied by a pale blue shirt and striped tie.

'No, the company issues it.'

'When I was in hospital I couldn't get used to all the uniforms. They've changed so since I was a girl. Ma was away in hospital for a hysterectomy in the fifties and the nurses then had super-starched aprons and white veils. They looked oh-so-smart with their big silver buckles on their belts. Now they're all dressed like shop-girls.'

'I like a woman in uniform,' Tom says. I glance across, daring him. 'In fact, Ruth often wears one at home, mainly in the kitchen.'

Our companions look uncertain.

'Just take no notice,' I say. 'He makes a lot of things up.'

All women know that tight skirts ride up when one is seated. Now the slit is well above my stocking tops and Reginald is seated next to the slit. I hope he doesn't view it as a come-on. His black outfit makes me think of an undertaker.

It is *haute cuisine* tonight and thankfully the half sea-sick tablet is now working. As a result, the wine kicks in more forcefully. I need to be alert in case I'm called. I don't want a passenger complaining that the doctor is drunk and incapable.

When it comes to the desserts, Pam, looking coy, asks Manas in a small voice, 'Could I try a little of each?' He returns with all four desserts on a large plate and down Pam's hatch they go. 'We always put on a stone when we go on cruises, but we take it off when we get home. Don't we, Derek?' Pam confides.

That easily? That inconsequentially? Should I warn them that they are both heading for diabetes; that's if they don't have it already?

Derek agrees. 'Yes. We bring larger clothes for the end of the cruise, don't we?'

Tom and I go off the idea of desserts. I decide to set a healthy example and order a single orange. The orange takes twenty minutes to arrive and is fridge-cold. I carry it around with me until we get back to the cabin. Five days later our cabin stewardess removes it.

In the bar the duo is playing. We take to the dancefloor. I can't move properly in the wretched tight black skirt, so I nip down to the cabin and change into a pair of comfortable black trousers and a top.

Back on the floor we let go in the rumba, *Rainy Days and Mondays*, eyes locked on each other, hips swinging in a succession of Cuban rocks and alemanas. Close together, we comment on our table companions with our lips pressed to each other's ears.

'God, isn't Reg a creep…!'

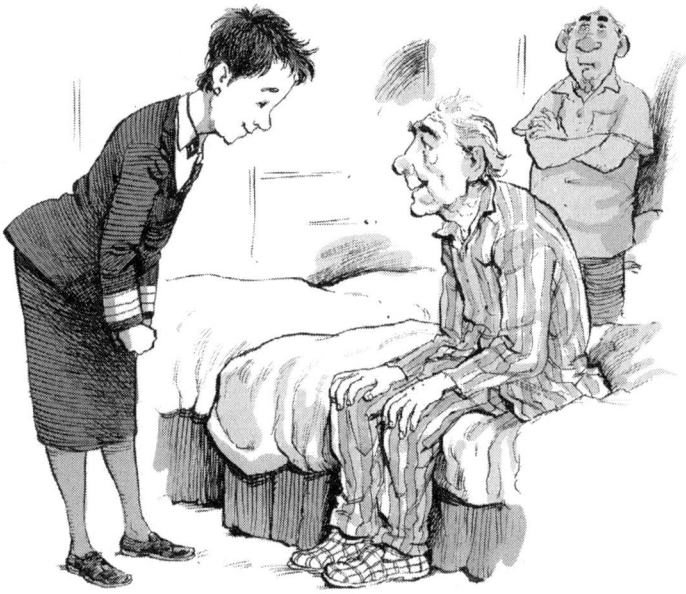

Day 3

Mr Armsure

Norovirus hitches a ride on cruise ships as they set sail in January for warmer climes. It is a common visitor to GP surgeries, where patients call it the Winter Vomiting Bug. The illness usually cures itself within a week but is highly contagious as well as dangerous in the frail elderly. It can be spread by the hands of unhygienic, unsuspecting patients for up to eight weeks – from A to B as Australians say – Arsehole to Breakfast.

Coralie looks up briefly. 'G'day, doc,' she says, then looks down at the patients' notes on the desk. Her dyed blonde hair is loosely tied back in a black rubber band, leaving the fringe dangling. She has thin but not unshapely lips, the top curling slightly over the bottom one.

'Where in Oz are you from, Coralie?' I sit on the chair next to the desk, normally reserved for a passenger, determined to break the ice.

'Sydney. I came aboard in Sydney. Did my training at Sydney Royal.' She takes stationery out of the filing cabinet ready for surgery and drops it down on the desk.

'Married?' I watch her movements, intrigued by the energy expended.

'Nah. I *was*. Didn't work out. I tell you – it's a mug's game.' She pulls a face.

'You must meet loads of men on board though.'

Coralie turns. 'Huh. *Them*. Nothing lasts in this place. Always saying goodbye.'

At a guess, from the lines on her forehead and neck, she'd be forty-five. But then, the furrows might be due to smoking, or stress.

'So, are you Sydney born and bred?'

'Yeah. North shore – Narrabeen. You know the Beach Boys' song, *Surfing USA*? Mum was brought up there. Never knew me dad. Mum kicked him out when I was a tiddler.'

'Narrabeen? We had friends there – Bob and Irene Dampf. Know them?'

'Nah.'

'Mum still there?'

'Yep. She's got another fella. But, aw, look, we don't see eye to eye. I steer clear of him most of the time.' She stops what she's doing and stares ahead.

'…so working on board must suit you.'

'Mm, I guess. But I'll've done ten years this year – too long. It's starting to get to me now, true. I mean, don't get me wrong, it's a great way of life, but… you know…' She sighs, shrugs her shoulders, then goes to the waiting room to fetch the first patient.

36

It doesn't occur to me that anyone working on board a luxury cruise ship could ever get fed up with it. My family's five voyages had been such stimulating adventures. A world apart. Ever changing scenes, ports and people to experience. A wonderland of discovery. As Ten Pound Poms (originally nicknamed by Australians as Prisoners of Mother England), we travelled out on the Assisted Passage Scheme with enthusiasm then returned to England in indecision. Later I found out the real reason for the boomerang voyages.

Dad used to assert that women were superior to men. His mother, who in 1912 had to marry his father because she was pregnant with Dad, was subjected to her husband's drunken, violent outbursts, so Dad grew up feeling sympathy for his mother and hostility towards his father. Dad was not only enamoured with women but craved their attention so much that one woman wasn't enough. I don't know when his affairs started but a number of our journeys were the result of Dad's infidelities. Mum attempted to control them by using distance as a cure. It didn't really work. For her part, Mum felt homesick for her mother, sister and four brothers, so she was keen to return to England.

⚓

The number of gastroenteritis patients increases. It is beginning to look like an epidemic. In our toilet-sized laboratory off the Medical Centre sits an innovative rapid testing kit for diagnosing norovirus. The instructions state that we need to collect at least ten patients' stool samples for the result to be valid. By day three we have enough samples and Coralie suggests that Liz and I do the tests together. Together? Is it so difficult that it requires two professionals to carry out a kit test? In fact, the instructions prove to be disconcertingly long-winded and complicated. You add diluent and activator to your sample, then you wait a set time until the next stage of mixing and setting aside. You mark time again before decanting your mixtures into special receptacles. In the final stage you set the stopwatch until you see a reaction and colour change. Everything has to be labelled so you don't lose track of whose sample is whose. It takes over two hours. Not to mention unpleasant. I won't go into it. No wonder Coralie has volunteered me and Liz.

One of the ten specimens proves strongly positive for norovirus. That explains why the illness is spreading so fast. But why not the other nine? Why don't they all test positive? A medical mystery.

'You'd better tell the captain,' Coralie advises.

'Really?'

'Yeah. He needs to know for the procedures.' She is emphatic. I ring the Bridge.

'Captain, we've got a positive noro test.'

'Are you sure?' The captain sounds displeased.

'Yes. We've just tested ten samples.'

'So, it's pretty conclusive. How many gastros are confined?'

'Twelve at present, but we've had four more this morning who we still have to visit.'

'Sixteen. And we are noro positive... so it sounds like we should bring in Code Orange.'

'Yes, I see,' I say, not knowing what Code Orange is, except that it isn't green, or red. It will be in the lever-arch file.

'You'll have to tell Dr Wallis too,' Coralie says.

'The doctor always does when there's an outbreak,' explains Liz.

Immediately a reply comes back: '*Bad luck. Send ten samples ashore to test for other pathogens and confirm noro. Enjoy the trip.*'

'Dr Wallis wants us to send off ten samples to confirm noro,' I call out, 'and check if there're any other bugs.'

'That's his stock answer. Look, it's a complete waste of our time. We never get any useful results, do we Liz?' Coralie says.

'Never. I've never seen any anyway,' Liz agrees.

'Still, we'd better do it, because he might ask us for the results. If we get a sample from every patient from now on we should have ten in a couple of days,' I say.

'Right, but we'll have to send them ashore in Madeira or Tenerife. Cape Verde'll be useless,' says Liz.

'I tell you what, let's send the ones you used for testing. That'd save us a lot of bother,' Coralie urges.

'They're too old. Anyway, we've chucked them, thank you very much.' Liz wrinkles her nose.

'The samples have to be fresh. But only liquid stools – don't send anything solid,' I elaborate.

Coralie looks at me, eyebrows raised. 'If you say so.'

At evening surgery Mr Wayfield returns.

'My cough's got a lot worse, doctor. It's keeping me and the wife awake at night. She's not getting any sleep, nor am I. Next door too, I wouldn't be surprised.'

I examine him. No fever. No wheeze. No chest noises. His peak flow reading for asthma is within normal limits. He assures me that he is using the cough mixture, boiled sweets and moisturising the cabin air.

'It's this air-conditioning. It just spreads the germs round and round the ship. I've heard other people walking round with the same cough.' Is he considering a claim against the company? I decide to ask the Senior Engineer about the air-con, so I have evidence-based information.

'Could you spend more time on deck, in the sea air?'

'In this cold wind?'

'Mm. Well. I can't find any sign of infection; no bronchitis,' I say in my best reassuring voice, 'and it doesn't seem to be your asthma,' Doctor Placebo says. 'So, I can't see any call for antibiotics.' Why do I put that idea into his head? Mr Wayfield looks fed up. 'Even though your peak flow reading is good, your breathing tubes are obviously irritated. I want you to try doubling up on your inhalers for a couple of days. Have you got them with you?'

'They're in the cabin.'

'If you need to come again, bring them with you and we can check your technique. In the meantime, see how you go with the inhalers, and come down if you need more supplies. If there are further problems, be sure to let me know,' I say and stand up, the signal that the consultation is at an end.

Coralie is on a coffee break. Liz does the billing. Surgery is over. I take the four new gastro case notes and set off.

Mr Armsure is a Yorkshireman in his late eighties. He is a retired engineer travelling with his friend, Harold Olroyd, also in his eighties, both sharing an inside cabin. No porthole. They and their wives had been friends for years when they used to travel together, until their wives died one after the other and the men decided to continue travelling in a twosome. Mr Armsure takes his time telling me the story.

'I don't think it can be owt,' he says, 'because I feel right enough. I would 'ave come down to t'spital but nurse said not to. I don't want to be a bother. I'm sure it's nowt. Harold 'ere made me report it.'

'Let the doctor *loo-ook* at you,' Harold stresses.

I examine Mr Armsure on his bunk and straighten up. He has Sheffield Umbilicus. As a Sheffield medical student, I learned the local wisdom that the umbilicus, or belly button, was your lifeline at birth and should never be messed with. Therefore, it was never cleaned, leading to a build-up of years of dark debris firmly stuck in its little trough. Quaint, but nothing to do with his gastroenteritis.

I don't like having such elderly patients tucked away in an inside cabin where I can't see what's going on, and from where they 'don't want to bother' me. It reminds me of an aged blind man I gave telephone advice to in the middle of a hectic norovirus outbreak in Newham when I first started working there. He must have passed a great deal of blood rather than diarrhoea. There was no way of knowing over the phone. It was two weeks later when he presented with severe anaemia and an obvious bowel cancer. He didn't survive long after the operation. I learned then that I couldn't know until I'd seen the patient for myself.

'Well, I'm very glad you did contact us because we've had a few upset stomachs on board, and we don't want the germs to spread.' Should I admit to having other cases? I've never worked for a private company before. Is it my responsibility to protect corporate reputation? 'Now stay put, Mr Armsure – you too Harold – until we give you the all-clear. You can order meals from cabin service – the telephone number is here.' I point to the directory sticker on their phone. 'Take plenty of clear drinks – except alcohol – and don't hesitate to let us know if you're worried about anything.' I give them instructions about contacting the nurse on call. 'We'll ring you ourselves in the morning. Any questions?'

'Could I go for a walk onto t'deck?' Mr Armsure asks, his head tilted to one side.

'Sorry. You have to stay put until forty-eight hours after your stomach's settled. That's the rule,' says Doctor Official-Policy.

Counting Mr Armsure, together with the other three cases, means that all four cases are confirmed. The numbers are multiplying.

Only one more day until we dock in Madeira. I am already longing to step onto solid, dry land. *Freedom.*

By morning Liz has attended another four cases, and two more are waiting to be seen.

I run up to the gastro meeting in the Senior Officers' headquarters next to the Bridge. Senior Officers from the ship's dozen departments are present. The captain presides, while his diminutive dark-haired secretary silently takes minutes on her notepad.

Without enough room at the central table to seat all the officers, the less prestigious heads of departments, such as bar, security and housekeeping, the non-Europeans, stand at the back of the room by the door.

Captain Strom starts the meeting. 'So, doctor, tell me: how many gastro passengers do we have now?' He looks at me and so do all the Senior Officers.

'Last night we had twenty. There's been four overnight, and there's two more to see this morning,' I venture.

'So, twenty-six?'

'I believe so.'

'And crew?'

'Oh, two crew.' I've forgotten about them.

'And you say we're noro positive?' The other officers suddenly pay attention. One or two murmur, a look of despondency spreading over their faces. They fidget.

'Yes. We tested ten samples yesterday and got a definite positive for norovirus.'

'Are you going to test any more samples?' I feel I am getting a grilling.

'We're sending them ashore for confirmation and to see if there are any other microbes responsible.'

'Are any passengers coming out today?'

'I'll check our list and let you know.' Why haven't Liz or Coralie warned me about the questions? They might have given me the stats before the meeting.

'So, do I take it that nought point two percent of passengers and crew are confined?' the captain is asking me.

'How many passengers and crew do we have?' I ask him.

'One thousand and eighty-two, altogether: seven hundred and fifty-seven passengers and three hundred and twenty-five crew. So, it's over zero point two percent.' Thankfully he does the calculation, while my mind whirrs like a liquidiser, spinning all my thoughts in different directions, fragmenting as they fly apart.

'Well, it looks like we'll have to bring in Code Red,' he says. Some of the officers groan and look at me.

'Do you agree? Code Red, Doctor? What is your opinion?'

'It's best to be on the safe side,' I offer, keen to get back and look up the lever-arch file.

'I'll leave you all to inform your departments. Any questions?'

'Can we run the dolphin race this afternoon?' Eric, the Cruise Director, wants to know.

'What do you think, Doctor?' asks Captain Strom.

How should I know? What is a dolphin race anyway?

'Just make sure everything is sanitised and it should be OK,' says Dr Educated-Guess.

I look up Code Red in the weighty ship's policies file: no buffet; all food and drink to be served by waiters wearing plastic gloves. The handrails and public areas are to be cleaned five times a day with double-strength chlorinated water. The jacuzzis will be emptied. All departments are to report cases of diarrhoea or vomiting to the Medical Centre. Cards for the bridge lessons are to be cleaned with antiseptic; books in the library too. Extra precautions, extra cleaning and a great deal of additional work for all the crew.

As I finish morning surgery Coralie announces that I have ten new cases to visit. *Ten.* She has admin to do and anyway needs a coffee break. With the gastro medical bag, mountains of plastic gloves and aprons, and my lucky blue stethoscope, I set off. Halfway down the corridor my stomach gripes and I start to sweat. I drop the equipment in an alcove and dash back to the cabin just in time for a turn-out. Oh no. Is it…? Remembering the company's definition, I reassure myself that one episode does not make a case. It has to be at least three. I drink water, wash my hands twice and step back into the passageway.

Picking up all the stuff, I wonder how on earth I'm going to get round ten cases. At least fifteen minutes in each cabin, maybe twenty, times ten. That makes at least *three hours*. And it is lunchtime right now. My stomach growls. I feel light-headed and very sorry for myself. Really, whose idea *was* this blooming trip?

I drag myself on. After an hour I've completed three cabins. Moving more and more like a two-toed sloth, I go back to the Medical Centre to fetch the blood pressure machine to examine the elderly passengers. My own blood pressure feels like I'm treading on it.

Coralie and Liz arrive back from lunch. I whine, 'I've only done three, and I haven't been to lunch yet,' putting on a pathetic face.

They look at each other with eyes-to-heaven expressions, then Coralie concedes. 'Orright. Give us the stuff. We'll do the rest.'

So, the doctor doesn't *have* to see the passengers to confirm the diagnosis. The nurses can do it. They'd done it during the night when they'd been on call, but I'd assumed that it must be my sole responsibility during the daytime. From now on I'm going to be more assertive. After all, there is only one of me. I comfort myself with the knowledge that we'll be in Madeira tomorrow. A reprieve from the toil. And land. Solid land.

A second episode of the gripes catches me and I speed to the cabin in time for another attack. I mustn't have a third episode or *I'll* be confined.

How would the ship manage without a doctor?

———⚓———

Meeting Tom in the dining room, I update him on the news.

'You look pale. I hope *you're* not getting ill. I'd find it very inconvenient,' he jokes. I diagnose a case of humour in bad taste. 'Well, listen to this… *I'm* lying on a deck lounger reading *Gone with the Wind* when a passenger comes up and stands very close, about where my knees are, and says, "You're the doctor's husband, aren't you?" I say, "Yes, but I'm not medical." She ignores that and says, "I don't want to bother the doctor – she's so busy – but I have this problem with my hip," and with that she lifts her dress up the side of her leg while I start to protest, "No, really, I don't know anything about this sort of thing" and I sort of throw my hands up in the air to try and stop her, and I'm saying, "No, no, you must go and see the doctor." She keeps saying, "No, no, I just want to…" so amongst all the "no, no"'s she flounces off totally dissatisfied. I bet she won't go anywhere near the Medical Centre – she won't want to spend the money.'

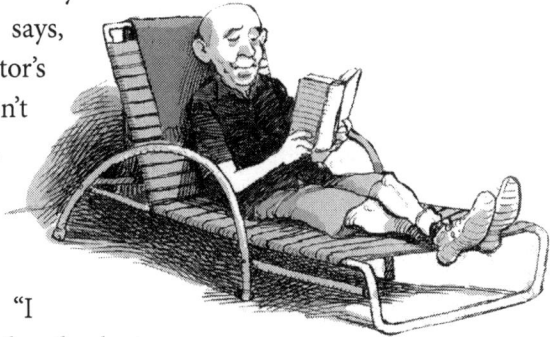

———⚓———

Liz, Coralie and I start the evening gastro calls early. Every patient confined to cabin is telephoned morning and evening. It takes ages.

'Is that Mr Armsure? It's Doctor. How are you doing this evening?'

'Oh, alright. I don't like being stuck in 'ere mind. I'm sure I'd be better wi' a breath o' fresh air. The air in 'ere just goes round and round. It can't be doing me a bit o' good.'

I can hear Harold, his cabin companion, in the background, shouting, 'The doctor doesn't want to know about *that*, Arthur. She's told you – you can't go out till you're better.'

They are both deaf, so are forced to shout at each other.

'But, how are you? Any more diarrhoea or vomiting?' I run through the questions.

'Well, I've been a few times.'

'*What for* – diarrhoea or vomiting?'

'No, I haven't vomited again.'

Harold is yelling, 'Yes you *did*. You don't remember – it were just after the doctor left.'

'Oh yes, I did once.'

'Any more diarrhoea?' I'm wishing I'd paid them a visit. It would have been a lot quicker.

'A few times.'

After failing to establish the precise number of episodes and timings for my record, I plead with Arthur to keep a tally, and promise to visit the next morning.

'Can I go ashore tomorrer then? Ee, I don't want to miss Madeira. It's the reason I've come on this trip. The wife and me had our 'oneymoon here in 1952. Ay, we did that…' There is a catch in his voice.

'I'm sorry, but there's no way you can go ashore. We have to view you as infectious and the Madeirans don't want infectious people wandering round their island spreading germs. I'm afraid you'll have to stay put, Mr Armsure. I'm coming to see you tomorrow. Are you getting room service?'

'Oh yes. I'm having fish and chips t'night. Champion.'

'If you've got an appetite that's a good sign, but I wouldn't have fried food if I were you. It's a bit hard for an upset stomach to digest. Stick to grilled or boiled. Anyway, I'll see you tomorrow.'

'Well, what can I have to eat then?'

'Choose something grilled or boiled – maybe with pasta, or rice.'

'I don't hold with that sort of thing, Doctor. I like to see meat and veg on me plate.'

'Do your best. I must press on now Mr Armsure. See you in the morning.'

If all the calls take this long, I'm never going to be finished in time for the end of the cruise, never mind evening surgery. I can hear Coralie and Liz in the background putting the phones down and picking them up, whizzing through the calls. No conversation, just, 'How many? What time? Stay put. Speak in the morning.'

There are now thirty-eight cases, all confined to cabin with their cabin companions.

According to Tom, someone said it was food poisoning from the lobster on Formal Night. Other passengers blame the air-conditioning and talk about eighty-three people being quarantined. Some are saying that the captain won't let us stop at Madeira to save the company mooring fees.

Instead of helping themselves to the buffet, passengers have to queue to be served. An air of discontent settles over the ship. Complaining passengers gather in small mutinous groups.

Evening surgery.

Angel, the receptionist we'd met on the first day, comes for her three-monthly contraceptive injection. Her husband works on board as a bar waiter. Coralie has gone for coffee and a smoke, so Liz takes Angel's blood pressure, weighs her and gives her the injection from stock. I wonder if Liz is contraception-trained. Her background is in accident and emergency. I make a mental note to ask. It might be important.

Mr Langford, a heavy-set man in his seventies, still with a determined head of thick white hair, and bushy eyebrows, ears and nostrils, attends for an INR (International Normalised Ratio), blood test to check blood thinning. He is taking warfarin to stop blood clots forming around a metal heart valve. We have an INR machine which Liz is expert at using so I am only too pleased to leave her to it. The result is ten point five – the highest I've ever seen. It is supposed to nestle between two point five and three.

'Well,' I say, trying not to drift up into an anxious soprano, 'your INR is actually very high today. It's ten point five. It's a good thing you came.' And by the way, I don't say, *Your risk of bleeding doubles with every INR point above three.* So, what's that, fourteen times the risk, or one hundred and twenty-eight times? Someone will know.

Mr Langford appears unconcerned, although he remarks, 'It's never been that high before,' and looks as if he is seeking an explanation, at the same time implying that it must be the medical profession's fault.

I run through his risk factors for haemorrhage, then his queries.

'Have you had any bleeding, or spontaneous bruising?'

'No, nothing. Will I get bleeding?' He looks surprised.

'Not necessarily.' Somehow I feel that if neither of us expect bleeding, he won't get any. So much for my expensive scientific training. After running through the possible causes of the high reading we move to his alcohol intake. 'What are you drinking and how much?'

'Um... a few beers during the day, and whiskies in the evening... oh, and wine with dinner.'

'More than at home?'

'Definitely more.'

I open the door to the office. 'Liz, have we got any vitamin K tablets?'

'Should have. Hang on.'

'Vitamin K is the antidote to warfarin,' I explain to Mr Langford. I don't add that it is essential for fertility in rats.

'I think I've been told that... greens, isn't it? My doctor says greens can counteract warfarin, so I suppose they'll have vitamin K, won't they?'

'Sorry, can't find it. Must have run out,' Liz calls out. 'No injectable either. I'll order some in Madeira if you do a prescription.'

'So, what you need to do, Mr Langford, is stop your warfarin now. It stays a long time in the blood, so come to see me after three days and we'll check your INR then. After Madeira we'll have vitamin K, if we need it. Can you moderate the alcohol?'

'But that's part of the whole pleasure of the cruise.'

'I see... then we'll just have to try and work around your drinking. But don't go to excess.' It will be fruitless trying to change Mr Langford's habits, especially on holiday. He might agree on the face of it, but then ignore my advice, leading to lies and needless conflict at the next visit.

Mr Langford smiles and nods. 'Sounds good enough to me, Doc.'

'And let me know, obviously, if you have any bleeding or worrying bruising. You'll be a bit more prone at present, so be careful,' says Dr Fingers-Crossed.

Liz does the billing. She shuts the clinic door with a bang and sinks into the chair by the desk. 'These gastros are a bugger, aren't they? We've got another three now.'

'No!'

'Don't worry. I'll see them after dinner.'

'Are you sure? Well, they're keeping us off the streets, but maybe now it'll ease up. P'r'aps we've reached a peak.'

We look at each other in silent prayer. Liz picks up the gastro log to fill in details of the new cases and adds the information online.

She looks very English. Like Liz Taylor. That pointed nose, sharp features softened by blue-green eyes, and pearly skin framing a trustworthy face.

'Where are you from, Liz?'

We are moving round each other, checking everything's been done, washing our hands, and putting things away. She is in blue scrubs with white shoes. Tiny feet. Must be size three. I bet she's a good dancer. We do the Tidying Tango.

'Sutton, in Surrey. Actually, it's Greater London now. Did my training at St Helier and St George's,' she calls out from the treatment room.

'I lived in Thames Ditton as a child, when we came back from Australia. Went to school there and worked in C and A's bargain basement in Kingston-upon-Thames on Saturdays when I was fourteen. I *loved* it. Fourteen and eleven pence a day. Subsidised canteen. We emigrated twice. Don't know how Dad wangled it. Powers of persuasion.'

'My Aunt was a Ten Pound Pom. I remember Mum and me waving her off at the docks in the 1970s. I was dying to go with her. It looked so exciting. That's what led me to work on ships.'

'It wasn't still going in the seventies, surely? I could have been a Ten Pound Pom three times!'

'It *was*. Till the 1980s. It was about seventy pounds by then.

Aunty Rose's sister, Ivy, went out with her, but she came back after two years. You had to stay for two years. Maybe that's how your dad did the scheme twice. Where did you train?'

'Sheffield. But I was twenty-six when I started medicine.'

'Twenty-six? What did you do before?' She stood still.

'I was a nurse.'

'*Really?*'

'Mmm. Adults and children – trained at the Royal Children's Hospital in Melbourne. When I worked with the doctors there I thought "I bet I can do that".'

'Aunty Rose lives in Melbourne. Rose Stannard?'

'Loads of people have relatives in Australia. Didn't over a million emigrate? How long've you been working on board?'

'This'll be my sixth year. I suppose I should think about packing it in.'

'Why?'

'Stuck in a rut. But it'd be really hard to get a job ashore now and I don't have a place of my own. All my stuff's at Mum's.'

'You could easily get agency work. You might need to take a refresher for certain sorts of nursing. I mean, at the moment there's a real call for nurse practitioners in general practice and it's a great job. Really varied. Good money too.' I sink into the patients' chair next to the desk.

'How much?' Liz eases into the seat behind the desk.

'Oh, about thirty-four thousand.'

'Really? But, don't get me wrong, I still enjoy the ships – well, not when there's noro, of course. It's a great social life. Have you always been in general practice?'

I talked about being an obstetrician and gynaecologist. 'But general practice was good for me actually because I started to get very anti-men, only hearing women's side of the story. Not that men haven't got a lot to answer for.'

'Tell me about it.'

Liz looked at her watch. 'Ooh, listen – I must dash. I said I'd meet Coralie at six.'

I feel on closer, more cordial terms with 'the girls'. That's all that was needed. A good natter. We'll be fine.

***

We must be out of the Bay of Biscay now as the ship is sailing so steadily it could be rolling on rubber tyres on a rubber road. I look out of the porthole. The sun has just set, leaving a dramatic red streak across the horizon, reflected in the sea. I stand stock still. It looks like the entrance to paradise. As I watch, the red glow fades, leaving an apricot flare high up into the clouds with a green tinge around the edges. Can the sky really be green?

***

'Another three cases,' I call out to Tom.

He appears in the bathroom doorway, drying himself with a white towel as big as a bed sheet. My glasses steam over.

'You're putting me on! I'm finding this very inconvenient. How many is that?' He steps down into the cabin.

'Over forty.' Water glugs down the plughole.

Tom complains about his visit to the gym, where a woman walked on the running machine for forty minutes. He says, 'Why doesn't she walk round the bleeding deck? The captain was on one of the other machines. He looks *very* fit. Good physique. He'll have been an athlete at one time, I'd say.' Tom, who was an athletic coach in his twenties, knows about these things.

***

After dinner we hook arms and go up to the Pool Bar where a

man is playing the piano and singing, a cross between Billy Joel and Elton John. Wavy brown hair, with a streak of grey over his right temple, and a white patch at the nape of his neck, like a stork mark. He rocks backwards and forwards rhythmically over the piano keys as he plays and sings. Coordination. Like patting your head and stroking your belly. Tom, a fanatical Bob Dylan fan, makes a request for *Heaven's Door*: a gentle jive. *Heaven's Door* feels just like it says on the tin. The cares of the day slide to the floor and are trampled.

In bed I lay reflecting on the strange society we find ourselves in, adrift, far from our familiar, comfortable civilisation. I see us as an abandoned tribe of deserters. We can behave anyhow in our isolated cocoon, our bobbing bubble, with only an empty sea stretching to the horizon. The world won't know what we're up to. Yet there are strict protocols and conventions to which we all unquestioningly, even devotedly, adhere. We'd dressed up that evening as though we belonged to an aristocracy, a ruling elite.

Why aren't we in grass skirts, boiler suits, or in the nude with body paint?

What stops us from descending into savagery as in *Lord of the Flies*? Will I resort to forcibly repatriating irritating passengers? Are we just slaves to the 'bread and circuses' principle of Juvenal, the Roman poet in the first century: as long as our stomachs are full and we are entertained, we remain placid, complying with the demands of the hierarchy? Those in charge and we who obey. Those on the Bridge and those below the waterline.

In the distance a bell sounds. And again. The phone is ringing.

'Hello Doc. It's reception. We haven't received the Port Health Declaration for Madeira.'

'What declaration?'

'Doctor, you need to fill out the Port Health Dec before we get to port.'

'But do *I* have to do it?'

'Yes, it must be signed by you and the captain before we get to port. We e-mailed it to you yesterday. There's a copy up here if you want to collect it.'

Damn. Damn. Damn.

I stare at the document. It demands to know if there is any infectious disease on board. *Of course there is an infectious disease on board.*

There isn't much that's more infectious than norovirus. Five virions swallowed from your fingertip can induce the illness. I stare at the lined page with its insistent columns demanding the names, dates of birth, cabin numbers, nationalities, dates of commencement of symptoms, and treatments for each affected passenger, and dates of release from quarantine 'during the voyage'. The *voyage*. That is *everyone* affected since *Southampton*, including those already discharged – over forty passengers in all.

Clumping back down to the Medical Centre, I bang the door closed and fetch the gastro log. I make up passengers' nationalities from the sound of their names as we don't include that information in the log. Besides, almost all of the passengers are Brits. I hope no-one will scrutinise it too closely. It takes over an hour to complete in legible handwriting. I am irritable. I feel fuzzy-headed from lack of sleep. Why didn't the nurses remind me? Why didn't I look at my e-mails? Oh yes. No time. This must never happen again. Health Dec completed and handed to reception I trudge back to bed in the dark cabin. It is two a.m. I set the alarm for six. I have to see Mr Armsure before surgery. Hell.

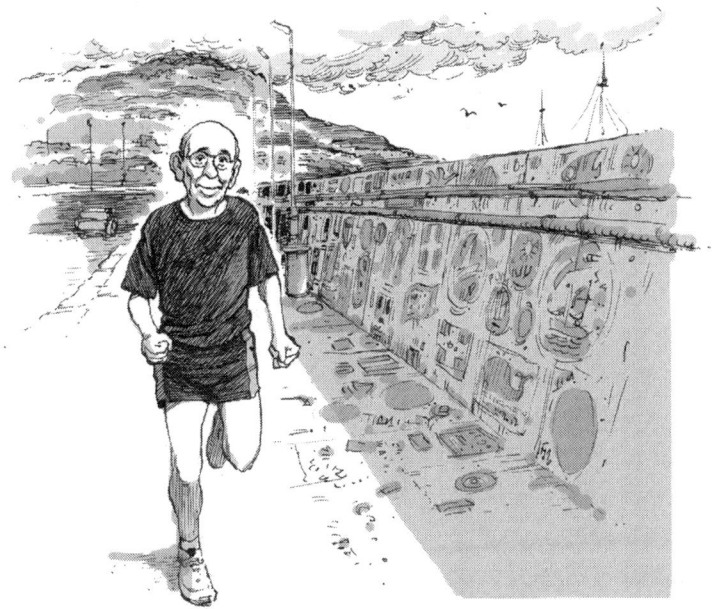

Day 4

Mrs Wilson

Mr Armsure is lying on his bunk in striped pyjamas. Harold is sitting on the edge beside him. Within a minute Mr Armsure, who was a structural engineer, is describing in technical detail the form, colour, consistency and dimensions of the stools he has passed since I'd spoken to him the previous night.

Harold interrupts, 'The doctor doesn't want to 'ear all that, Albert. She just wants *the number*, don't you, Doctor? Just *tell 'er the number*, Albert.'

After some debate as to whether a repeat visit immediately after leaving the toilet counts as one or two episodes, Harold and Albert decide the total amounts to five.

This does not sound good. Here is a man in his late eighties, in a place where I can't keep a close eye on him, continuing to have multiple episodes of diarrhoea. Thankfully he has no vomiting and minimal abdominal pain, but is he getting dehydrated or low blood potassium, which he is losing in the diarrhoea? I have no way of knowing. There aren't facilities to check on board. I'd have to send his blood ashore and wait an unknown length of time to receive the result, by which time his potassium level will have changed. His blood pressure is on the low side. From his moist-enough tongue and reasonable skin turgor he doesn't appear dehydrated, but they aren't reliable indicators. He has passed urine, so his kidneys are still functioning. Not that I want to wait until they aren't.

Hearing the scraping sounds and feeling the bumps of the ship docking at Funchal, Madeira, I feel a fillip of excitement in my solar plexus, like a waking creature stirring.

'I'm sure I'd be better wi' some fresh air, Doc. Can't I just walk round the deck? I wouldn't even touch owt. It'd just tek ten minutes,' says Albert.

I am only too aware that he and Harold are confined to an inside cabin with no porthole. I feel claustrophobic in the cabin and I don't suffer from claustrophobia.

'Sorry. Not possible, Mr Armsure. I've said, once you're confined you can't leave until we give you the all-clear. The bug is highly infectious and we don't want it to spread.'

Harold adds loudly, 'She's already *told* you that, you *can't go out.* No good asking.'

Albert is not impressed. 'I know, I know. What is it then, *this boog?*'

I explain about norovirus. 'Has housekeeping been to clean your cabin?'

'They have that, lass. A right gang of 'em came yesterday, all got up, wi' space suits and masks and all. You'd think it were the plague in 'ere. Ee, 'ave you been to Eyam, lass – in Derbyshire – the plague village?'

'Yes. But I have to say, the sanitation team would draw the

line at washing your money in vinegar and handing it through a porthole. Anyway, I must get on. Let us know if there are any worries – if you're worse, start vomiting, or have any questions. I'll see you this evening. Drink plenty of clear fluids – anything you can see the bottom of the glass through, except whisky.'

Harold laughs politely. I don't think Albert hears.

'You've got three passengers and two crew outside,' Coralie says as I turn into the Medical Centre fifteen minutes late. I know. I've just walked through the waiting area.

Two unrelated passengers attend with swollen ankles; another has conjunctivitis. The two crew members are there for repeats of contraceptive pills.

During surgery I can hear Coralie banging objects around in the office as I take my time seeing passengers and crew. Then she rings the gastro patients: 'How many times? Stay put. We'll ring tonight.'

A man appears at the office door dressed in casual clothes. He smiles. 'Morning. I'm Sergio – Port Agent. You've got a prescription for me?'

'Here,' says Coralie, picking up the envelope from the desk and handing it to him, with barely an acknowledgment. Coralie is ill-tempered, again.

'Thanks. See you later then. About four?'

'No later. We leave at four-thirty,' Coralie announces.

'OK, see you then,' says Sergio, unperturbed.

Liz arrives to help with the gastro calls. Coralie goes for a coffee break.

After surgery I ask the nurses about the Port Health Declaration. I tell them about getting up in the middle of the night to complete all the passengers' details.

'*What?*' Liz's eyes widen. 'But I sent the log to reception before I went off!'

'You mean reception had the info *all the time?*'

'*Of course.* We always e-mail them the log before we get to port – the night before. It's standard. All the gastros are on the computer anyway. They've got access to the log and they just have to attach it to the Health Dec and fill in the nationalities. They've *got* all that stuff. Trouble is, they say it's not *their* job, and we say it's not *ours*. But that's bloody unacceptable – getting you up in the night for it.'

'Right. Then we need to get this sorted. Who do I contact?'

'Dr Wallis is your man. E-mail him,' says Coralie. 'None of us should have to fill out the Health Dec. We're up to our armpits with noro. I'm telling you: lazy buggers, the whole flaming mob o' them. *God's oath.*'

Seven short blasts and one long toll on the ship's alarm. Eric, the Cruise Director, announces, 'Proceed to your muster stations,' meaning it is crew lifeboat drill.

I run back to the cabin for my lifejacket, then dash up five flights of stairs. Gasping at the top, I wonder how far I am from the nearest life support machine. I'm on the wrong deck but the lifeboats are even-numbered on one side and odd-numbered on the other, so I scoot across to the opposite side of the ship and run down one deck to locate lifeboat five. My companions are already standing in a straggly line. The boatswain is shouting out the crews' numbers. 'One-nine-two!'

'Here!' I croak, red-faced and panting.

We spend a lot of time standing around whilst crew attendance is checked and verified by two-way radio with the Chief Officer on the Bridge. But it is *warm*. Warm with a balmy breeze. The sun, which I've barely seen since Southampton, is shining hotly on my skin. The air smells tropical; the light shimmers. Looking ashore I can see palm trees waving by a children's playground and Madeira's jagged green mountains looming over the island. How heavenly it looks. I can't wait to go ashore.

My bleeper sounds.

I walk to the nearest phone.

'Security. We have a Mr Armsure at the gangplank, cabin three-one-four, says he's going ashore but he's down on the confinement list. Has he been released?'

'No. He certainly has *not* been released. He's not allowed to go ashore. Can you please send him back to his cabin.' Muttering follows.

'He says he wants to speak with *you*.'

'*I'm in the middle of drill.*'

'Can you just speak to him?'

'Hello Doc. Ah only want to walk out on t'shore. Only walk. It's where we 'ad our 'oneymoon. I promise I won't touch owt. It's for t' memory of my Edith.'

He sounds so pathetic, so small and desperate, I want to be Dr Kindness and say, '*Yes, of course you can, Albert. You go on then.*'

Instead, I am Dr Company-Regulations, saying, 'There's no way, Mr Armsure. You're not better yet, and you're infectious. When you're in isolation you have to stay put until you're discharged. I'm sorry. This is all you'll see of Madeira today. You'll have to go back to your cabin.'

'Are you sure I couldn't just touch the land and come back? I'd be ever so quick. Honest I would.'

'Mr Armsure, your security pass has been cancelled, so you wouldn't be able to get ashore anyway. Sorry. I *am* sorry. Put the security officer back on the phone, will you? I'll see you tonight.'

Back at the lifeboat station three crewmen start the operational procedure to lower the boat into the water. Chief Officer Tallak is moving along the deck observing the crew's performance, stopping here and there to examine their knowledge on technical questions.

At the next lifeboat a small group of crewmen gather around the bow amidst a hum of masculine consternation. One manoeuvre is tried over and again, producing a clanging sound but no movement. Tallak investigates. A multitude of frustrated grumbling can be heard in Filipino and English. In the end, number seven lifeboat is not launched.

Ours hits the water, the motor roars, it circumnavigates the ship and then is hauled back up into its davits, dripping rivulets of seawater across the deck.

The tannoy crackles into life. 'This is the captain from the navigational bridge. Would all Senior Officers report to the Bridge for debriefing.'

I am a Senior Officer, so this means me. Drat it. More delay. What am I going to learn from, or contribute to, a lifeboat drill debriefing?

On the Bridge I become aware that all the other officers are in cream summer uniforms whilst I am in navy blue. Why haven't I been told? Oh – those blasted e-mails. You'd think Coralie or Liz might have said something. I feel uncomfortable on the Bridge. Don't have the right uniform. Nothing for me to say.

'Two crewmen were asleep in their cabins – two-eight-seven and two-two-six. They had to be woken. I warned them it will be a disciplinary matter if it happens again,' the Security Officer, Kikato, informs Captain Strom.

The Hotel Manager whispers to me, 'No tropical uniform?'

'Tailor hasn't got my size,' I lie. 'Alterations.'

Captain Strom is saying, 'I expect the crew to set their alarms so they attend drill when they've been on night duty.' He looks around to nods of assent.

'One of the lashing hooks jammed on lifeboat seven and couldn't be freed. It might need an overhaul. The deck department will try servicing it in place, but if that doesn't do it, one of the engineers will take a look.' This is from the Chief Engineer, Sergei.

'Could you see which part? The screw or the hook?' asks the captain.

'Can't tell right now.'

'So, it must be freed and tested before the next general emergency drill. Put it on the agenda for the next meeting,' the captain addresses his secretary, who stands behind him, slightly to one side, with her notebook and pen. Short and as slight as a wraith, I don't notice her presence until now. I imagine her as a sea nymph, beautiful, in flowing robes riding a seahorse.

My legs ache. I suppress a yawn.

I run down to the cabin. Tom is sitting on the sofa flicking through the guidebook.

'Have to see the tailor first.'

'Don't be long,' Tom calls out as I let the door bang.

Dayap's door is locked. The laundry men, ever-occupied, are taking whites out of the massive washing machines, steam-rolling sheets and hanging ironed uniforms onto racks in departmental order.

'Do you know where Dayap is?' I ask Gabriel, the laundry manager.

'Gone for lunch,' he answers without looking round.

'When will he be back?'

'About four.'

Four? Too late to get a new uniform. Surgery starts at five.

Dayap knows my size. I write a message, which I push under

his door, asking him to bleep me if there is a problem with supplying the cream uniform today.

With such a sense of relief that it takes me by surprise, Tom and I walk down the gangplank onto firm, dry land.

The sun is in its rightful place above the island instead of drifting across the ocean. I fill my lungs with what feels like the first oxygen in four days as if it was a lifesaving reflex. Then the harbour wall hits me in the eye. I stop, jaw slack. 'Did you see this when you ran round the port?'

Tom has medals for middle-distance running and was determined to run around each port while I finished surgery.

Two hundred metres long, the wall is layered in graffiti and murals from top to bottom. Colourful paintings of boats with names and dates tumble into each other, with images of sailors, female figures and foreign script: a pictorial maritime history.

'That? It's been done by sailors landing here over the years – centuries probably,' Tom says. 'The crews did the artwork to congratulate themselves because it was the first port they came to and it was dangerous crossing the Atlantic. Some of them were in a race so were boasting of their win.'

'How do you know?'

'Guidebook,' Tom says.

Like two swells we stroll along the promenade, drinking in the normality of everyday life in Madeira, away from the regimented systems on board. Ship life is the ultimate in freedom for those who don't have to work at sea. We step on the startling black and white mosaic paving stones depicting anchors, crabs and fish. They enliven my feet. I am on a glorious vacation for two and a half hours, away from the ship's illnesses and isolation. Time to explore and to eat out in peace, beyond the range of my tyrannical twenty-four-hour bleep, sometimes referred to in hospital as *the albatross* from *The Rime of the Ancient Mariner* by Samuel Taylor Coleridge in 1798. The mariner shot the ship's escorting albatross, which the crew hung round the mariner's neck. It became the ever-present curse of the voyage.

The dazzling sunshine casts everything into sharp relief and the air smells foreign and aromatic. People are going about their daily lives just as they must have done all the time that we were out at sea. Young couples sit on the sea wall drinking cans of fizzy pop while watching the waves roll in. Parents amble the length of the front with excitable and fractious children, stopping under the shade of each violet-flowered jacaranda tree. Chic elders, nattily dressed in autumnal colours, carry shopping baskets and an air of purpose. Towering above us soar Madeira's dizzying, jungle-clad mountains, capped in floating clouds.

Pigeons, with their staccato walks and bobbing heads, search the ground for crumbs, comfortingly indistinguishable from those in Trafalgar Square. Why do they bob their heads with every step? I'll look it up when I get home.

'There's a market in the guidebook... somewhere...' Tom knows that I look for them wherever we go. It is a piece of social research: what the local produce is; whether the place is packed or empty; what people are buying; whether the earthy stallholders doing gritty jobs are chirpy or worn out – a barometer of the local economy. And retail therapy, of course, an opportunity to buy something unusual that we won't find at home. A chance for Tom to get his fix of avocados, to which he is addicted.

He scrutinises the map, navigating us up steep side turnings, through car parks and past municipal bins until there it is: the Mercado dos Lavradores, the Farmer's Market.

I've never seen so many bird-of-paradise flowers, flocking together in zinc water buckets. They look as if they'll take a peck out of your arm as soon as look at you. If only I could take the pineapples, guavas, herbs, and raw sheep's milk cheeses back to our cabin. Back to England. The avocados are bright green and huge. Tom carries away a bagful.

From the bottom step of the basement the pungent smell of fish envelops us, clinging to our clothes and hair. Draped over white marble slabs with their long, pointed tails and heads of needle-sharp teeth lay row upon row of unrecognisable black eel-like fish looking as though they've all been run over by the same steamroller. Huge blue-tiled illustrations of market life from a previous century decorate the walls with scenes of long-gone street sellers wearing strange skull-caps with top-knots. They must have carried their baskets of wares on their heads. Today canny locals and curious cruise-ship passengers mill around the stalls.

A restaurant two doors down from the market looks like someone's front room. The restaurateur, who resembles one of my uncles, speaks English and recommends the local fish: the squashed eel from the market. Tom looks it up in our guidebook, reporting that it is called a scabbard. It makes us laugh out loud even though it isn't funny. I feel my shoulders drop back to their natural position under the shadow of Madeira's prehistoric laurel forests hugging its tall volcanic peaks.

Tom knows that I love facts. Scientific, solid and certain. 'I bet you didn't know that Madeira came out of the sea eighteen million years ago. You'll probably remember that…'

'*Thank you.*'

'…and what about this – only four percent of it is above the waterline. It's the largest underwater mountain in Europe.'

'No kidding.'

'I'm telling you. But there's more. It's actually sinking into the sea under its own weight.'

'Ah, but that's alright,' I say. 'We won't have so far to get back to the ship after we've eaten our own weight in food.' We agree that the sinking of Madeira is in our favour and laugh again. I drain the two-gulp coffee cup.

'Give me the guidebook,' I say. Tom chews all his food fifty times while I bolt mine as a result of years of bleep-disturbed meals whilst a junior doctor. I flick to some photos of small creamy-coloured carvings. 'Hey now, look at this. They have scrimshaw here. Scrimshaw.'

'I've heard of it, but I couldn't tell you what it is, if that makes sense.'

'Yes, you do know. They're those ivory carvings done by whalers. They used whale bones and teeth and walrus tusks. Walruses in Funchal? Give over!... Anyway. If we see one, let's get it, shall we? Even the name is great – *scrimshaw*. Sounds like a Yorkshire policeman. Constable Eric Scrimshaw reporting for duty, sir. Eh-oop, lad.' I laugh. Tom doesn't.

There is no meal better than fresh fish just cooked and what with sautéed potatoes and a glass of ice-cold wine for Tom (I'd fall over if I had wine in my enfeebled state) it feels like the best meal we've had for days. Like eating a Madeiran mama's cooking. Mentally I tuck away the memory for another time; maybe a birthday surprise one day.

'We'll have to come back here for a proper holiday, don't you think?' I hint.

'Mm, if you like,' Tom says between chews.

I feel disappointed that Tom doesn't entirely share my spirit of adventure. He'd been a nervous evacuated war child, leaving him with separation anxiety and the desire for a secure environment. I was post-war. It made a difference. As a Ten Pound Pom with a restless father, I'd been travelling since I was two years old. As Daddy's girl I'd acquired his wanderlust, his urge not to miss out on any of the wonders of the world. I can imagine that Dad might have been an intrepid sailor in the 1700s, criss-crossing the globe, exploring newly found lands and keeping a log of his experiences. Now I was taking over his imagined role.

Our two-and-a-half-hour holiday is fast disappearing as the sun and Madeira sink into the sea. Tom stops in front of a small jewellery store. 'Wouldn't that be one of those things... errh... grimshaws? Look – there. There!'

All I can see are dolls dressed as nuns.

'Oh yes, the sailing ship. *So intricate*. But look – eighty-two euros. That's a bit steep. Well, if it's still here next time we come, I'll buy it.'

On board, deck-hands wearing blue latex gloves are chlorinating the banisters.

My cream uniform hasn't arrived.

'Three more gastros,' says Liz.

Will this epidemic never end?

I visit Albert and Harold.

'What were you thinking of, going along to the gangplank, Mr Armsure?' I ask, raising my eyebrows for maximum effect. 'Don't you remember, I told you, you couldn't get off while you're in quarantine?' I raise my voice. 'You shouldn't have been out of your cabin at all,' says Dr Do-As-I-Say.

'Yes, Doc, I know, but I reckoned, for my Edith, it'd do no harm to just touch the shore.' His voice drops.

Dr Forgiving relents.

Albert gives me the daily report. Things are improving at last, although Harold disputes the number of stools as well as what Albert is eating.

'I told you, you shouldn't 'ave had them chips at your lunch. You 'ad a right to-do after that,' Harold reprimands.

'No, I didn't.'

'You did.'

Why was room service providing gastro patients with chips? Especially as norovirus can cause temporary fat intolerance. I'll have to raise it with the chef. The ship needs a gastro diet. Something light. Something white. In a 1958 domestic science lesson, I'd had to prepare a meal for an invalid. It consisted of steamed potatoes, steamed fish and steamed cabbage. Colour-free. There isn't actual medical evidence to show that any particular diet makes a difference to the outcome of gastro; but I ask you, *chips*? Still, I don't have to worry about Mr Armsure now. He is definitely on the mend if he feels well enough to eat chips.

In the Medical Centre Coralie is on duty.

'Liz 'n' I did the gastro calls while you were out,' Coralie clips.

'That's great. Thanks. I've been up to three-one-four checking Mr Armsure. Anyway…' sensing she doesn't want to hear about Albert, I say, 'how was your day, Coralie? Did you get ashore?' and reach for the gastro log.

'Yep, just a coupla hours. I always go to one of the cafés on the square and get the local wine. White and very cold. Alvarinho. A real good 'un. A tonic. You should try it. I love it.'

'Sounds nice. Just you?' I scan her face.

'Yeah. The others – you know, Marion from the shop, Val, and all of that lot – they went to the hypermarket out of town. I don't need any of their stuff. Dead boring.'

I smell the wine heavy on her breath. Would she have drunk a whole bottle on her own, or more?

'Mr Langford's waiting. His INR's in the notes. Here… oops.' She drops the notes, grunting as she bends to pick them up.

I'm not due to see Mr Langford until tomorrow.

'I've got a big bruise on my shin, so I thought you'd want to see it. You said report any bruises. But really, I know how I got it. It was on the edge of a trolley in the supermarket, so I know where it's come from.' As usual he looks unconcerned.

'Is it painful?'

'Only if I press it.' I was more interested in painless spontaneous bruising in his case, but still, I had said…

'Is it getting bigger?'

'Let me see…' he pulls up his trouser leg and scrutinises it. 'No-o, I don't think so. Oh, I don't know… it might have spread down here a bit.' He points to the purple lower end of the contusion just above his ankle.

'It's probably tracking down. Gravity. It looks like it's going to form a blood blister. But just leave it to its own devices. If it breaks let the nurse know and she'll dress it. Nothing elsewhere?'

'Not that I've noticed.' Bruises in unexposed places are more relevant. We knock ourselves a dozen times a day on exposed parts of the body, unexpectedly finding a bruise on a hip or elbow. We don't knock ourselves in our armpits.

'Good. Your INR is nine point seven today. Coming down. Hang on. We might have vitamin K…' I open the consulting room door.

'Nurse, did the port agent bring vitamin K?'

'Couldn't get it,' Coralie calls back.

'Ah… Well, keep off your warfarin then, and come to see me in three days; unless there's anything worrying you in between time.'

Worrying *him*? Three more days for me to keep my fingers crossed. I decide to check our stocks of intravenous blood substitutes as soon as I have the chance, to reassure myself that we are ready if Mr Langford haemorrhages.

'You've got three passengers waiting and a crew member,' Coralie growls after Mr Langford leaves, blowing a short sigh through pursed lips. I get the message. Hurry up.

Another passenger has the Ship's Cough.

Someone who'd fallen in Funchal wants to check that nothing is broken. All accidents, whether on ship or shore, have to be recorded on a comprehensive set of accident forms signed by the doctor and the passenger and sent to the Safety Officer, with a copy to the Chief Officer. Was the passenger wearing appropriate footwear? Was the passenger under the influence of alcohol? Were they on a shore excursion? The company wants to ascertain liability. It all takes a long time – the form-filling, the examination, the advice, the treatment, and the associated discussion.

A woman suffering from headaches is next. Teasing out the cause of recurrent headache and examining for potentially serious diagnoses is never a quick consultation with a new patient. Mrs Wilson is in her sixties, of heavy build with a florid complexion. She is on diabetic and blood pressure medication. I take her blood pressure. It is sky high. Stroke high. Two hundred and ten over one hundred and seventeen.

'Mrs Wilson, have you been taking your blood pressure pills regularly?'

Something falls with a clatter outside. Coralie curses and I hear a scraping sound. We both look in the direction of the sound.

'Never miss. First thing. I've always done it. Always. When I get up, first thing.' She is matter-of-fact. 'I haven't missed any. Why, Doctor? Is my pressure up?' She frowns.

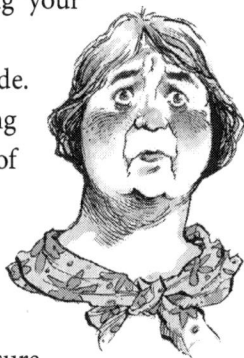

'Yes, it's very high at the moment. That might be why you're getting these headaches – although I have to say – it's not common to get headaches with blood pressure.' Would she reach the door without having a stroke?

'I'll do it again in a few minutes to double check. It might start coming down now you've been sitting for a bit. Any leg swelling or breathlessness?'

'Actually, my ankles *have* swollen up on board, but I've not taken that much notice. They always do. And I'm not any more breathless than usual. I don't think so. No.'

I press her ankles and sound her chest. Her puffy feet indent to the pressure of my thumb, but only up to the ankle bone. The second blood pressure reading is slightly lower than the first, but still too high. Would she get to her cabin before having a stroke?

'Has your diet changed on board? Have you put on weight?' A nasty question.

'Oh, I expect so. I eat more. Can't help it. There's so much lovely food. And with the buffet – well, you just keep helping yourself… I have to say, though, some of it is too salty for me. I hardly use salt at home nowadays. My doctor said not to. But I suppose I must've put on weight because my clothes feel tighter.' She pulls at her shorts' waistband, which has sunk between the rolls.

'That will probably be why your blood pressure is up. Hop on the scales.' I pull them out from under the couch.

'Oh *no*. Do I *have* to?'

'It'd be useful to have a baseline. Let's see… eighty-seven kilos. That's thirteen and a half stone in old money,' I say, referring to the conversion chart on the wall.

'Oh, I'm usually about thirteen. *No* – don't say I've put on half a stone. Already!' She looks satisfyingly shocked. I shouldn't have to talk to her about diet now.

I take a third reading. Slightly lower again, but not enough to be safe. 'It's come down a bit with rest, but it's still too high. One hundred and eighty over one hundred and ten. You'll need to double up on your blood pressure pills for the time being.' Would she have time to take an extra pill before having a stroke?

Should I have warned her not to exert herself?

I arrange to see her after three days, if she survives.

The noises from outside my consulting room become more noticeable, as well as Coralie's impatient responses to telephone calls. I overhear her snap 'I can't help that!' in a raised voice followed by a sharp click. 'Have you finished?' Coralie asks as I open the door. I catch the whiff of alcohol again.

In General Practice I'd learned to smell patients' alcoholic fumes between the door and my desk. I even came to recognise whether it was last night's or that morning's drink.

'Yes, it's just the billing now.' I sound as normal as I can, but I resent her tone. I should tackle her right away, but it always takes me three days to think of how best to put my thoughts and feelings into words when there is a potential conflict.

Coralie is looking down at the billing documents. 'Cabin number?' she snaps at Mrs Wilson, finishing the process like an automaton. Mrs Wilson leaves and I listen to her footsteps receding. No thud.

I go to collect the crewman from the waiting area. His problem is a chronic irritating rash – urticaria. He's struggled with it for two years and is having a miserable time with generalised itching and wheals. Luckily, I did a six-month hospital job in dermatology so feel comfortable managing it. I explain the condition and the skin care, prescribing him antihistamines and skin creams. Other medications are an option, I say, if things don't settle. He is to return for review in a week, or sooner if worse.

By the time I finish it is obvious from Coralie's face and irritable movements that she is in a thoroughly bad mood. I feel distinctly uncomfortable as she barely speaks to me and avoids eye contact, while jamming stationery and equipment untidily into drawers and cupboards. She disappears into the treatment room, where it sounds as though she is practising the timpani with oxygen cylinders. It is a relief when Liz arrives to take her to dinner.

In the refuge of our cabin, I step out of my uniform and flop onto the bed.

When Tom wakes me, my new cream uniform is hanging on a hook on the wall by the cabin door. Was it there before and I hadn't noticed it, or has one of the crew members crept in whilst I was sleeping? The tailor or the laundry crew must have master keys.

By the time we arrive in the dining room our table companions are quaffing their wine and discussing the day.

'Och, we had a marvellous time!' says Mary. 'Ye go up to a place called Monte-something on the cable car and in a minute you're away from the top in a wicker basket. Two men jamp on the back, kicking off like on a scooter, skittering round the bends. So fast! Such a thrill!' Mary grins. I haven't seen her smile before. This is anxious, hypochondriac Mary speaking, her back-combed hairdo bobbing.

'Aye – it reminds me of when I was a wee bairn and ma da made a cart on wheels. It was a fearsome thing.' Jim is animated, for him.

'Ah, but did ye no see the dolphins? All jumping out the water right by the ship,' says Mary.

'When?' I ask.

'Oh… now, around seven in the morning. Just before seven. We were after walking about the deck, watching the ship come in.'

'*Oh no.* I was visiting a cabin. If I'd walked out on deck, I'd have caught them. I'd *love* to see some sea life. As far as I can tell there's nothing in the sea.'

Derek pauses over his steak and chips. 'Did anyone go to Reid's? We got a cab up there for afternoon tea. We booked it before we left home not to miss it. We've been before, haven't we, Pam? We knew it would be good.'

'They do a delicious afternoon tea. The hotel is gorgeous

– old-fashioned – all dark wood and heavy curtains. And it overlooks the sea, doesn't it, Derek?'

'I'll say. Right up on the cliffs. Terrific view. Must be America next stop.'

'Or Morocco. Depends which way you're looking,' Tom says.

Derek gives Tom a look. 'But anyway… they've got a beautiful pool on the terrace – one of those infinity pools. Some of the guests took their bathers with them. We didn't want to swim though – not after a meal.'

'You know, loads of stars have stayed at Reid's,' Pam says. 'Winston Churchill. Who else, Derek?'

'Oh, George Bernard Shaw… um… Scott of the Antarctic – all those sort of people,' Derek looks vague.

'So, what was it like?' I ask. I can't imagine it being superior to the ship's afternoon tea with its extensive range of biscuits, fancy cakes, sandwiches and scones, which I'd seen passengers carrying piled high on small plates on my way to surgery.

'Oh, they have everything – biscuits, cakes, sandwiches. What else, Derek?'

'Scones, lots of different jams and cream. Fresh fruit. Loads of special teas and coffees. Much as you want. You can keep helping yourself. And you can order wine.'

'Sounds great. I'd love it,' I say, hoping Tom will take note.

'Now see what you've done,' Tom teases. 'She'll be wanting to go to Reid's next.' I give him an encouraging smile and nod.

'And you, Reg?' Tom asks, leaning across me. A strand of Reg's sculptured hair has fallen down by his left ear. Should I say something?

'I'm not a scones man, but I don't have to tell you that Madeira's the place for wine-tasting. Downtown there's a shop that specialises in Madeira wine. Near the town wall. I got six bottles to take home, but would you believe it, they took every one off me at security. I won't get them back until Rio. I was looking forward to a tipple in the cabin.' Reginald purses his lips.

'Obviously that's why they take them off you,' says Tom. 'They want you to buy the ship's booze. If everyone brought their own, they wouldn't sell the stuff on board, would they? They'd have to charge you to use their glasses, or five pounds for the peanuts.' The social scientist is speaking. I knee Tom under the table.

'I daresay. Well anyway,' Reginald continues, making his small snorting noise in the back of his throat, 'it was in a sort of wine cellar, in the old part of town, with stone walls. There were these pumpkins hanging from the ceiling, all different shapes.'

'Gourds,' says Mary.

'And I can tell you,' Reginald continues, 'the owners there know what they're about. The lady gave me a plate of these small cinnamon biscuits to go with the Madeira. Tiny. One bite. I polished off the lot. And best of it was I didn't have to pay for them. But I nearly missed the boat on the way back – they were just pulling up the gangplank.'

The matter of Bush threatening to attack Iraq and Blair's complicity arises. Pam thinks it's sabre-rattling. I report that a soldier patient of mine has already been sent to the Gulf in preparation for the war.

⚓

Tom and I run up two decks to the Pool Bar. As we look round for a seat, I notice Liz at a table near the back, her head bent towards the singer with the brown wavy hair. They are in intimate conversation. That's quick work. Or maybe they already knew each other from a previous cruise.

The duo is playing *Top of the World*, the old Drifters' song, to the beat of Carrie's jingling tambourine as she strikes it hard on her thigh. The next number is *Honesty*, by Billy Joel. Tom and I do a 'Why Dance'. In close hold we sway slightly and Tom makes up the steps, which take us nowhere. Pressed close together and hardly speaking or moving – why dance?

Dad had invented the *Why Dance* when the whole family took to the dancefloor in 1962 on P&O's S.S. *Fairstar* sailing to Australia. We teenagers had taken lessons in ballroom dancing from the age of thirteen. It was the route to the opposite sex. Dad took up tap dancing aged seventy. The whole family loved to dance and Dad's *Why Dance* was a comic, ironic label he invented.

Dave and Carrie play *Please Mr Postman*, knowing we will honour them with a swinging jive, arms and heels beating the rhythm. We catch our reflections in the floor-to-ceiling windows, through which a string of lights from the Bridge to the bow of the ship shine and swing against the black night.

Three dance hosts, in their bright white trousers and navy blazers with shiny brass buttons, amble into the Pool Bar and sit with a group of unaccompanied women. Eleanor is tall and slender, with large grey eyes, an Eastern European face and a relaxed manner. She is a mechanical engineer, a shop steward. Unmarried. Edward, one of the younger dance hosts, six feet tall, with neatly combed salt and pepper hair, a surgical scar on his left cheek, and an easy smile, has taken a fancy to Eleanor and dances with her as much as he can get away with. Regulations state that affairs with the passengers are strictly forbidden, according to one of the dance hosts.

When Tom jives, women's heads turn. It is his most lively dance, in which he has perfected an alluring knee-knocking routine among half a dozen other moves. Eleanor pleads with him to jive with her. He demurs, then agrees. Two jives later he escorts Eleanor back to her seat and drops down next to me.

Peter, the oldest-looking dance host – who is sportily lean, wears fashionable rimless glasses and speaks with a speech impediment, making an R sound like a W – asks me to dance. We swing off into a silver medal foxtrot to *Baby It's Cold Outside*, the duo sounding like Dean Martin and Doris Day who sang it so beguilingly in 1944. *Divine.* We chat about this and that, comparing notes on Madeira. Tom doesn't know the slow foxtrot and I can only do it with a very good lead. Peter is that lead. As he steers me back to my place I can tell from Tom's long face and dumb stare that he is not pleased. I know why but I pretend not to notice. WORDS will have to be spoken.

The duo prepares for their break, introducing the brown-haired solo singer as 'the talented maestro, Lee Marsden'. Extracting himself from Liz's company, he walks over to the grand piano on the stage and plays a rumba. Not many people dance rumba, so Tom and I are first on the floor, feeling like a cabaret act. We've learned a great routine at dance school so we show it off. The dance hosts and their charges follow, some getting away with a social foxtrot. Slow-slow-quick-quick-slow. It fits the rumba beat. Next is Elton John's *Crocodile Rock*. Finishing with a flurry of stamping and spinning, we head down to the cabin.

'Did you really *mind* me dancing with the dance host?' I confront Tom as soon as we are out of earshot of the bar. 'You had such a *look* on your face when I sat down…' I stare ahead, thin-lipped.

'Well, *I* don't want to dance with anyone but you, and I thought *you* wouldn't want to dance with anyone but me.' We walk to the stairs as though we are strangers.

'*Come on*. Are you honestly saying I can't dance with someone like the dance host, who is totally proper and does dances you can't even *do*? Women ask *you* to dance and I have to watch you flirting and playing up to *them*.' We stop arguing to let a passenger go past.

'I was *not* flirting. *Do me a favour.*'

'You *were*. You should see your body language. You did your knee-knocking-mating-ritual smiling into that woman's face. You should *see* yourself!'

'Alright. I won't dance with anyone else. That's it!' Tom sets his face.

'I'm not *saying* don't dance with anyone else. You can dance with whoever you like; besides, it seems churlish to say "no" if you're asked. But I'm not putting up with you flirting in front of me!' We pause again as we pass a group of passengers, nodding our 'good evenings' as if everything is fine.

Tom was a war baby. At the age of three years he was sent away from the east London bombing to Tooting Hospital for six weeks to allow his mother to recover from the birth of his sister. Two years later he was admitted to Bishop Stortford Hospital for a further six weeks due to pneumonia. Parental visits were discouraged – so as 'not to upset the child'. Separation trauma had left its mark, leading to the desire for attention and the making of strong attachments. I had my own attachment issues due to my parents' unstable relationship.

'*And*,' Tom says thrusting his hand into his jacket pocket for the door key, 'I want to be asked first.'

'Then you ask me too. *OK?… Deal?*' We reach the cabin.

'Mm,' Tom grunts, not looking happy. We are supposed to be happy.

It brings to mind a photograph of Mum and Dad at the dining room table on board P&O's S.S. *Strathmore* in 1952. A white-coated waiter is bending over the table, serving Dad from a large silver tureen. Dad is looking across the room vacantly, maybe into the distance, maybe at someone on another table. Mum is confronting the camera with a look that says 'Has it come to this?' My brother David is trying to smile. I'm hanging my head and look sad. Dad's infidelities and the associated rows and silences made us all feel unsettled. Mum and Dad stayed together 'for the sake of the children'.

—⚓—

Waking up with a start, I check the bedside clock. 2.15. Hell. Thoughts about Coralie clatter round inside my head. Tom, the trade unionist, has advised a disciplinary. 'Coralie, I want to speak to you… Coralie, come in here please… Coralie, can I have a word?'

I feel nervous about the meeting. The anxiety and the endless mental rehearsing make me toss and turn. After all, I'm not even her employer. What if she explodes or slashes me with a scalpel? Worse still, what if nothing changes? What then?

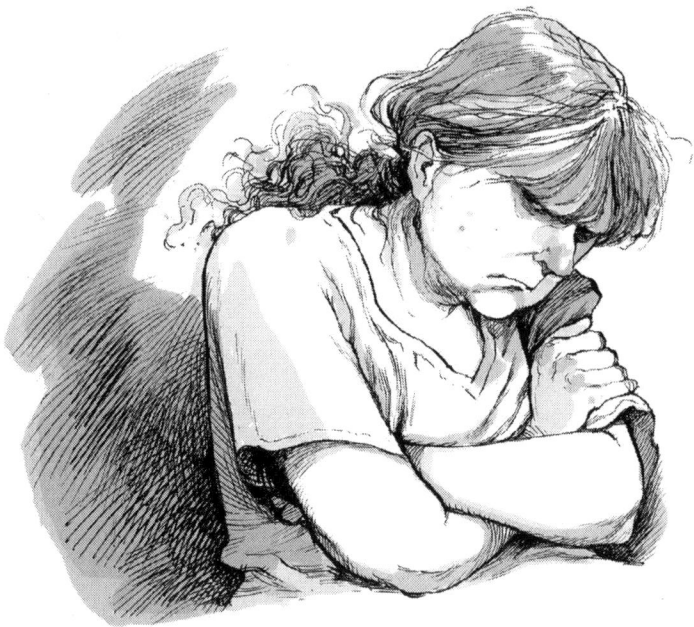

Day 5

Mr Langford

Coralie is already in the Medical Centre.

'Morning,' I say. 'Sleep alright?'

I try to behave normally, but the tension in my shoulders makes my neck ache.

Mr Wayfield is back. He sits down hard in the chair next to my desk. 'This cough's still there. It can't keep going on like this. The inhalers haven't helped one bit. Someone's got to do something. It's just going on and on. You must have *something* for it. My doctor gives me antibiotics when it's like this. Even the people in the next cabin are complaining.'

'Let's see then. Any fever?'

'No.'

'Any phlegm, or wheeze?'

'You asked me the same questions two days ago. *No.* The

point is, what are you going to give me?' He breathes out hard.

'Have you brought in your inhalers?'

'Yes. Here.' He takes them out of his pocket and thumps them down on the desk.

'Show me how you use your inhalers in a minute. Just let me have a proper look at you first.'

Mr Wayfield screws up his mouth.

'Deep breath.' My examination reveals nothing new.

To demonstrate the asthma test I stand up and blow out forcefully through the breathing apparatus. A musical squeak of air escapes from my bottom. The last patient I want to humiliate myself in front of is Mr Wayfield. He looks at the peak flow metre. I hope that he thinks the noise came from the equipment. Neither of us say anything as I feel my face burn. I pass him the hand-held device, saying, 'Now you.' He might have copied me blowing air from both ends, but doesn't. The metre reading is within normal limits. My face cools. Mr Wayfield sits.

'Good. Let's see you use your inhaler now.'

He puts the inhaler to his lips and presses the top twice, inhaling deeply. Some of the vapour escapes from his nose and more from the corners of his mouth.

I remind him of the correct way to get the best out of the inhaler. 'Stand up so you get your full chest expansion.' Men like Mr Wayfield like to think of themselves as having a big capacity.

Mr Wayfield puffs out his chest and sucks in the vapour.

'That's much better. Your chest should feel the benefit within forty-eight hours. I tell you what – I'll write in your notes that you can collect a prescription for antibiotics without needing to see me if you don't feel you're making progress after two days,' I say, even though I feel antibiotics are not only futile but over-prescribing and probably adding to the global antibiotic resistance crisis. The plan buys us some time at least, and if the antibiotics do work – well, stranger things have happened. 'But it's worth improving your inhaler technique first. It's certainly worth a try.' I'm sorry that I said 'try'. It doesn't imbue confidence.

'So, what do I do if that doesn't work? *Eh*? What if I'm no better?' Mr Wayfield glares.

Two other passengers attend with the Ship's Cough. One is diabetic with a fever and noises in her chest, so I have to prescribe antibiotics. Pity she really needs them. I anticipate Mr Wayfield will find out before she gets back to her cabin.

I push my door ajar.

'Come in please, Coralie,' I say, my voice rock steady. Or do I shout, '*Coralie, you get your arse in here now.*' She slouches in wearing blue scrubs a size too big for her and sits down in the patient's chair, glancing at me from under her fringe.

I remind myself of the Assertiveness Training techniques I'd learned in order to manage a difficult father. I know what to say.

'Coralie, when you've had a drink... I don't know if you know this, Coralie, I don't know if you're aware...' My voice rises and I stretch myself up to full seated height. I'm long in the body. Coralie looks at me, leans back and folds her arms. 'I don't know if you realise this,' I continue, planting my feet, 'but when you've had a drink – like yesterday, for instance... you know, when you got back from the port, you said you'd drunk that wine in Madeira, I don't know if it was a whole bottle or maybe more – anyway, when you've been drinking your behaviour changes.' My mouth feels dry. Or maybe I spat out, '*What did you think you were bloody well doing drinking a whole vat of wine in Madeira? Drink is a bleeding curse, Coralie. And it makes you the frigging devil.*'

'Wadja mean? No, it doesn't,' Coralie snaps, 'a coupla drinks isn't going to make any difference to *me*.' I assume then that she's a habitual drinker.

I moisten my lips. 'Well, *I* notice a difference.' That's straight out of Assertiveness Training. Tell them the effect on *you* – they can't deny it. 'You definitely changed. I mean, you were banging things down, making a lot of noise. You were impatient, short with the passengers, irritable with me. Made me feel very uncomfortable.' Or perhaps I said, '*You drunken soak, Coralie! You keep that up and you'll be out of here like a runny stool. You've been a monumental pain in the bum. Now just pack it in or else...*' 'Or else' – stage two of the disciplinary process straight out of naval disciplinary procedures in the Age of Sail 1550–1850 is twelve lashes with the cat o' nine tails. If she strikes me, she'll be hanged from the yard arm.

'You don't know what you're talking about. It wasn't like that at all. You've got that all wrong.' She stares me out.

'Well, it *was* like that from where *I* was sitting. That's how it was to *me*.' Coralie makes a face and looks away. 'So, if you're coming on duty, I don't want you drinking beforehand. OK, Coralie?'

'Whatever,' she says. 'Is that *it*?'

'Yes. That's *it*, for now.'

She gets up, exhales through puffed lips and leaves the door wide open.

I'm relieved that *it* has gone pretty well, although if there was to be a mutiny and I was elected captain I'd have her lashed to the mast. That would definitely be *it*.

My Melbourne high school motto was *potens sui* – self-control. I feel pleased that I've maintained self-control, externally at any rate. Inside I'm shaking.

Confrontation is difficult. It had been a regular feature of Mum and Dad's relationship. Dad's affairs led to stormy arguments that would rock the household with tears from Mum, thunderous shouting from both of them and door-slamming, followed by days of silence. It is an emotional legacy that, after the disciplinary, makes me feel as though I have a deep hollow in my solar plexus filled with lead.

At the gathering of the chiefs in the gastro meeting I report, 'Three discharged, four new cases. A total of forty-two in confinement.'

Captain Strom asks my advice about his noon report. It's the daily announcement of the weather, the ship's position and performance, and any notices. It's an ancient convention. In the days of sail the naval day ran from midday to midday. Noon was the easiest time to measure by the sun's position before sea clocks became weather-proof in the eighteenth century.

'How much attention do you want me to give to the hygiene side? I don't want to make it a big issue for the passengers,' he says.

'The passengers already know there's a gastro outbreak, so the more advice about hand-washing the better. Also not touching things – handrails, handshaking and so on. And I've seen people avoiding the hand disinfectant at the entrance to the dining room,' I say, glad to be able to feed back an observation that can be acted upon.

'We can't tell passengers not to hold the handrails. We'll have more accidents,' Captain Strom says, looking across the table. 'Oleg – can you make sure the boys give *everyone* the hand cleanser?'

'Yes, they're already doing it,' says Oleg, the Hotel Manager.

'The trouble is that passengers in electric wheelchairs hold on to their handlebars and drive right through,' says the Maître d', Arvin, standing very straight at the back of the room.

'So, the dining room boys must stop them,' says the captain. 'I'll say something about it in the noon report. Anything else?'

There follows a discussion about the cabin stewardesses reporting signs of stomach upsets to the Medical Centre. The meeting is over.

I catch the Chief Engineer. 'Sergei, I want to ask about the air-conditioning. The passengers with coughs say it's due to germs being recirculated round the ship through the air-conditioning ducts. Can that be right?' Sergei is tall. I crick my neck to look up at him.

'No, no. There are air vents that draw in the air – sea air – that's all. No recirculating.'

'But where are the vents?'

'All round the ship. You go up to deck eleven and you'll see them on the side panels. Thirty-six of them.' Sergei is moving slowly towards the door.

'And where does the air go to?' I keep alongside him.

'It just comes *into the ship*.' He runs his fingers through his hair.

'But what about the cabins?'

'The same.'

'So, it comes in, then just drifts out? Are there filters?'

'Yes, of course. All the air vents have filters. They're checked every week, and replaced once a month.'

'Ah. And are they tested for bacteria, for microbes?'

'Sure.' Sergei's answers are getting shorter. 'Regularly.' His bleep goes off. 'Sorry', he says, looking at the bleep's visual display, 'got to go.'

I find Tom on deck at a table in the shade, where he's spread out his mini pots of watercolours and is using a drawing pen on a thick sketch pad. An old mauve toilet bag he keeps his art gear in lies on its side in the sun, the contents spilling onto the table.

'How are you getting on?' I look at his sketch.

'I don't know whether this bit should be blue or purple.'

I squint at the drawing with one eye. 'Mm, black. It needs a small black square right here.'

After retirement Tom took a Fine Art degree. His speciality is abstraction.

'How about your day?'

As I tell Tom about the disciplinary with Coralie in a hushed voice, I shift my cadaveric white legs into the warm sunshine and hitch my skirt above my knees. The sparkling azure ocean is swishing by. The day is balmy. A warm breeze touches my cheek. I long to sit there for all eternity.

The deck scene reminds me of a photo of Mum when, in 1949, like many other British Jews, she took the opportunity to emigrate to Australia with Dad and us two children, as far away from memories of war and the Holocaust as possible. Mum is lounging on a deckchair snappily dressed in striped shorts, dangling equally pale legs, espadrilles tied around slim ankles. She would sit discussing politics with London friends in Yiddish, a language she grew up with. Mum and I were both gigglers. We could laugh at things that weren't even funny, like a spillage in the kitchen, or a dress caught on a rose thorn. Her friends would ask her 'Wus lakhst du?' Why are you laughing? It was a question Mum used to demand of me when I shook with snorting sniggers as a teenager. Now, Yiddish terms such as *nosh*, *schlep* and *chutzpah* are part of common parlance. With Dad a comic and Mum laughing so readily, they made a congenial match early in their relationship.

Passengers are gathering at the handrail on the port side. It can mean only one thing – a sighting. We rush over.

'Someone saw a whale spouting... Over there.' A woman waves her hand in the direction of the ocean.

We stare, intently scanning the waves, questioning any sign of life – shadows, ripples, spray, a breaker, spouting – but no. Nothing. We move away.

In the 1950s there always seemed to be a whale following the ship, and a great wandering albatross with its ten-foot wingspan gliding above the funnel in the updraft. Perhaps it was because the ship threw out leftover food into the ocean. Now it's all liquified and discharged into the watery depths.

At evening surgery Coralie doesn't appear. Liz is on duty. The disciplinary isn't mentioned. There is an e-mail from the Safety Officer, Ramon, about compulsory Safety Training the next day when we are due to dock in Tenerife. Pain. Will I never get a whole day in port?

In the Pool Bar that evening I tell Tom about the training. He groans.

'Again? You did it in Madeira.'

'No. That was lifeboat drill. One day we'll get the whole day ashore.' We agree that Tom will run round Tenerife in the morning and find a decent café for a scrumptious cappuccino.

He's been a serious runner since the age of eighteen, winning cups for mile races and county competitions. He'd even been offered an athletics scholarship to Colorado State University after coming second in inter-county championships, but his parents had dismissed the idea. Being working class, they'd insisted that he would be better off finishing his six-year apprenticeship as a hand compositor in the printing trade. It would stand him in good stead for the future. Still, he'd kept running in competitions and for pleasure ever since. We arrange to meet back on board, then go ashore for our two-and-a-half-hour holiday.

'Did you go to the port talk?' I ask.

'Not very inspiring. I could get more from the guidebook. In fact, it sounded like he was *reading* from the guidebook. I think it was one of the officers – no, I tell you who it was. It was that man from the tours desk. The tall blond one – you know the one I mean? Seven feet tall. He sits there with the dark-haired woman. I think he's Danish, or Swedish. I'm not sure. We're probably related, with me being from Viking stock.' This was one of Tom's favourite jokes, his looks rather resembling one of the shorter, skinnier, balding, black-haired Vikings. 'I was none the wiser when I left the talk, except that there's going to be some sort of festival in Santa Cruz. Whether it's religious or more like Notting Hill Carnival, search me. But it was weird – he kept saying Tenerif-eh, which got very irritating. Tenerif-eh,' Tom mimicked him. 'Try to get off early, will you?'

Lee Marsden is playing *Goodbye Norma Jean* by Elton John. A gorgeous, slow rumba. I drag Tom onto the floor. I can't wait to dance. Once on the floor I forget everything. Time stands still. It is just Tom, me and the music.

Now a waltz. All the dance hosts stream onto the floor with their partners. Everyone knows the waltz. Tom isn't keen. Too old-fashioned. 'Come on. Let's try our whisk and weave,' I urge him.

'*What*? How do we do *that*? Oh *no*. Do we *have* to?' He looks panic-stricken.

We circle the floor twice before we feel ready for the move, asking each other which foot to start on and whether to place it behind or in front of the other. It's a tricky manoeuvre. I give the instructions in Tom's ear. We get it completely wrong and collapse into hooting hysterics, causing annoyed couples to collide with us. After apologies and composing ourselves, we set off once more. This time we crack it without even thinking and feel smug. To prove it we do it again, and again.

~⚓~

The phone rings in the dark cabin. Not the Health Dec, surely? I feel cross. Liz is speaking. 'Can you come and see the man in six-nine-nine? He has severe abdominal pain. You've seen him before – Mr Langford.'

'Coming.'

Mr Langford is writhing, holding his left side and grimacing. He looks pale. Liz is standing beside him with the blood pressure machine in her hand.

'What happened?'

'I don't know,' he gasps. 'I just went to the toilet,' he puffs. 'When I came back, the pain started,' he pants. 'It's got worse.' He screws up his eyes and rocks his body from side to side.

In his abdomen a huge tense, tender lump occupies his left side, the size of a football. Nothing that I have ever read about in a medical textbook.

'You've had a bleed,' I say, my heart beating faster.

'You said I might...' he groans.

It is five-thirty a.m. In the Medical Centre we put in two intravenous lines, one in each arm. We give him blood substitute. No vitamin K. Has the bleeding stopped? Could he exsanguinate? I have no idea. We have to keep his blood pressure up with intravenous fluids and get him to hospital – fast. I tell Mr Langford.

'What then?' he grunts.

'They'll give you vitamin K first. Then they'll do a scan to see the extent of the bleed and where it's coming from, and decide what to do next.' I use surgical first principles. It is a completely unfamiliar scenario.

I give Mr Langford a small dose of morphine, then ring the Bridge and explain that we need to disembark our patient via ambulance urgently, immediately the ship docks. Could they get a move on? Possibly. Sailing faster means greater fuel consumption, more company expense. The ship uses fifty gallons of diesel oil per mile as it is – one gallon for twelve feet. We are due in at seven a.m. Tenerife is not far off.

The sound of the ship's engine takes on a different register.

Liz arranges for housekeeping to pack up Mr Langford's cabin. An e-mail goes off to the port agent, to Dr Wallis, copied to the captain and all the departmental managers. Liz telephones the port agent to book the ambulance and arrange the hospital admission. She fills out pages of repatriation forms. I contact Mr Langford's insurance company.

'Do you want me to ring someone at home?' I ask.

'I suppose – my son.' He looks fearful and suddenly older.

His pulse and blood pressure hold. I'm banking on the force of the pool of blood pressing on the leaking blood vessel to stop further bleeding.

We dock at six-thirty with a clunking sound and a jolt. I look out of the porthole. The ambulance is on the dockside. The ambulance crew bring in their stretcher. Liz and I see Mr Langford down the gangplank and into the ambulance with his luggage.

'I hope you go on alright,' I say, squeezing his hand. I'm sorry to see him go. I wonder if he will sue the company, or the Medical Department, or me, because we lacked vitamin K on board.

Liz and I don't say much at breakfast.

'That's me done for,' she says, leaning back in her chair and dropping her head on her chest. 'Still,' she looks up, 'I'll stagger ashore. Got to stand on dry land.'

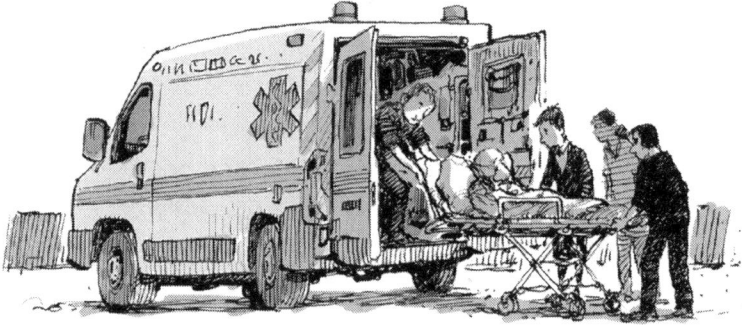

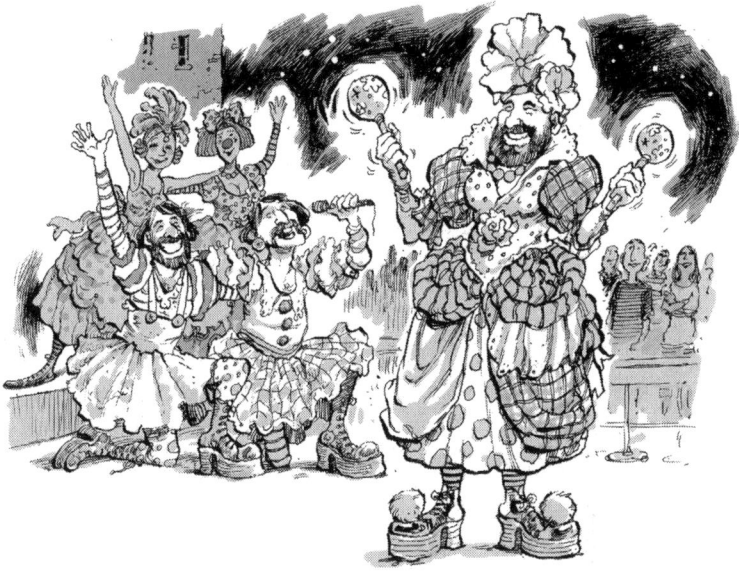

Day 6

Mr Wilson

The Medical Centre is deathly quiet. I think about Mr Langford and all my other charges, mostly elderly, at high risk medically. Basically, my job is to keep them fit enough to celebrate their final years, to make sure they don't die on board, to keep the association of pleasure and suffering well apart. After all, once you're over thirty-five, your chances of dying before the draw are greater than of winning the National Lottery. Your odds turn from being a winner to the risk of becoming a loser. I am here to prevent my passengers from losing their bets.

Checking all the bleach-reeking rooms, it is clear that Coralie hasn't been here. One of the nurses is always in early to start the watertesting, a routine chore to check the bacterial levels in the pools and jacuzzis, after which they start ringing the gastros. At eight o'clock I open the doors. On my own I get patients to complete their details on a proforma. Surely Coralie hasn't got the surgery opening time wrong. She knows very well it is earlier on port days than on sea days. Or is she seeing a new gastro patient, or an emergency in a cabin? No message.

'And now the painful part – the billing. Forty-five pounds for the consultation, plus the medication. Nurse'll work it out when she gets back, then it'll go on to your on-board account.' The passengers sign an incomplete invoice. I remain studiously ignorant of the electronic payment procedure. I don't want to know.

A woman rings. 'Can I get out now? I've been in the cabin for four days. Nurse said if I was OK, I could leave today.' In the background I hear a male voice saying, 'Tell 'er you're going ashore.'

I check her entry in the gastro log. 'Any symptoms?'

'No. I'm absolutely fine. Honestly. Can I please get out?'

'Yes, as soon as you're ready. The sanitation team will fumigate your cabin. You'll need to be out for at least three-quarters of an hour. I'll get your security card unlocked.'

I confirm her discharge to all departments.

Still no nurse. I ring the nurses' on-call bleep. No response.

The phone rings again. 'Anton, Second Engineer here. I'm waiting for the water testing results. Are they ready?'

'Nurse is tied up – sorry. I'll tell her you're waiting.'

'When will we get them?'

'As soon as she can finish them.'

I ring reception for Coralie's cabin number, then call her.

'Hello.' A gravelly voice.

'Coralie? Shouldn't you be in surgery?'

'Ah, er… What's the time?'

'Ten past nine.'

At nine-thirty Coralie comes in, just as I'm closing the doors.

'Did you oversleep?' I try to sound casual, but there's a steely edge to my voice.

'Must have.' No eye contact.

'I bleeped you but you didn't answer. That was the on-call bleep. What if it was an emergency?'

'Ah, yeah, sometimes it doesn't sound in the cabin. Best to ring.'

An emergency bleep that doesn't function in an emergency?

'Anton rang. He's after the water tests.'

'*Christ!*'

She grabs the equipment and dashes out, slamming the door.

I start ringing the gastros. Forty-two of them. Forty-two times three equals one hundred and twenty-six. Two hours and six minutes.

It is nearly ten o'clock. Right. I start with the ones due for release today so they can go ashore. Coralie will have to take over the remainder. That's all there is to it. As my Yorkshire midwife friend, Ann, used to say: 'Let that be an end to it.'

The bell rings from the waiting room. We are closed.

'Yes?' I peer out through the crack in the door.

'Morning, Doctor. I've come to collect the samples.'

'What samples? And you are…?'

'Marcus. Tenerife Port Agent. I was asked to come and collect samples for the laboratory between nine and ten, and a prescription.' He looks too young to be a port agent. To be out in long trousers.

'Samples? Oh, yes. Stool samples. Just a minute. Come in.' I widen the crack.

In the sample fridge there are six stool pots. None are bagged up and all are without request forms. No time to do them.

'Sorry, Marcus, they're not ready. Can you come back later?'

'I don't think so. I've got three ships in today. I'll be busy all day. I'll come back with your prescription, but that will be at the end of the day.'

'But if you find time later, would you ring us?'

He strokes his chin. '*If* I have time.'

'Hang on.' I hand Marcus an envelope. 'Prescription.'

I scrawl a note to Coralie: '*Port agent samples not ready. Need bagging & forms. Will ring later if he has time to collect. Rang few gastros – see log. Training now. Billing to do for pax.*'

⚓

In the below-decks metal training room an assortment of crew sit in departmental groups, each in their distinctive uniforms. On the deck above, passengers are strolling ashore into the sun and climbing into their tour coaches. Some crew chat, some lounge, others, in jeans and t-shirts, yawn and doze in the grey windowless room. Those with their eyes open stare at me as I sit near the front. The Safety Officer, Ramon, stands beside his PowerPoint presentation. I haaa on my glasses and clean them on the hem of my skirt.

The slides flick from one to the next while Ramon reads them out, with occasional ad libs in a solemn voice: 'It is forbidden to throw anything over the side – *ever*. Most important – lit cigarettes. The wind can carry them back on the decks and start a fire. Code Bravo is the alarm code for fire. Code Bravo training will take place on the voyage. The fire extinguishers are marked by these symbols, here… and here.' Ramon taps the photographs of extinguishers with his white pointer. 'You will receive training. Before the training, look up the manual. Where are the training manuals?' He looks around the room. Two or three crew mutter while I try to look as if I know the answer but don't want to show up the others. 'Yes, these are situated in the Officer's Mess and Crew Dayroom. Water extinguisher is for paper and wood, carbon dioxide extinguisher for electrics…'

It is hypnotic.

'And finally...'

I jerk awake.

'What do you do if you see someone acting suspiciously?' Ramon stares into the group. Crew shuffle in their seats. I try to look like I am giving the others a chance.

Silence.

'You report it to *me*, or to the *Bridge*. Ring reception and ask to bleep me, or ring the Bridge telephone. Do not try to tackle the situation yourself.' The presentation is over. I collect my certificate.

'You should *see* it, darling. *Un*believable!' Tom has caught the sun.

'You ran round?' I throw off my uniform.

'*Ran*? You are joking. No-one could run out there for a start off. Spent most of my time walking round with my mouth open. There's lots of big hairy men, ten foot tall with beards, dressed in weird women's gear.'

I brush my teeth, spraying foam on the mirror.

'They're part of this festival – expressing their femininity, no doubt. Who knows? It's all along the promenade by the port. *Totally packed*. Masses of families with kids. And not only cross-dressing-men – the women are also outrageous. You've just *got* to see it. *Come on*.'

Carnival arrived in the Canary Islands with the fifteenth-century conquest of the archipelago by the Spanish. Tenerife, off the coast of Africa, is in the middle of the trade route between Spain and Latin America. The result is a carnival with influences from all three cultures. Extravagant feather headdresses derive from African societies. A unique modern event is the Marcarita Ponte Tacón, the Men's Marathon in High Heels, entertainingly resulting in broken heels, twisted ankles and tumbles. No Health and Safety here.

A joyful mayhem greets us as we step out onto the extensive Santa Cruz esplanade. Thousands of people mill around featuring, just as Tom had said, big men dressed incongruously in garish women's clothes over false breasts. Their fluorescent blue eyeshadow, rouged cheeks and red lips, hairy legs and huge feet all conspire to produce an appearance of barely contained lunacy. No-one stares, except us. No-one picks a fight. The atmosphere is the essence of tolerant communion. The men's imaginative costumes are startling. Dressed as hula-hula girls, some have squeezed into grass skirts, sporting green wigs at jaunty angles. There are clowns with painted faces and orange hair, spacemen wearing Perspex bubble helmets and moon boots, supermen in scarlet underpants over blue leotards, seventeenth-century grand dames, some masked, in beaded crinolines and tall wigs topped by mounds of plastic fruit.

The women wear hooped skirts with huge feather headdresses; clowns' outfits with white woolly wigs, striped pantaloons and elongated red clowns' shoes. Some in scanty glittery bikinis show off their buttock cheeks, bulging boldly either side of a G-string.

Adults swing squealing children round by their arms. Other youngsters are chasing each other, hopping on one foot, or licking multicoloured lollies. Parents look relaxed, confident that their children are safe and if lost, will be found. The excitement is infectious.

Bands of musicians stand in the square playing loud conga music, tapping their feet to the beat. Huge posters of someone called Celia Cruz, entitled the 'Queen of Salsa', adorn billboards. In an extravagant full-length silver gown, the bodice edged with exotic grey feathers, her brown face is larger than life, eyes live as hot coals.

The main square, Plaza de Espagnol, on the front, has been constructed to look like a village, above which Celia Cruz's name is illuminated in blue neon lights. A young couple is dancing a quick, hip-flicking Cuban salsa; she is in a kingfisher blue figure-hugging dress that, Marilyn Monroe-style, swings out to expose her athletic legs and black knickers; her partner looks dashing in a bandana, flamboyantly tossing his black curls at every spin.

In a café on a small covered terrace overlooking the square, the waiter seats us at a long table on the end of a bench. Our neighbours look like locals. They glance at us and we nod a pale English greeting. 'It looks like a Cuban theme,' I deduce from the programme on the table, using school-girl French and conjecture to make sense of the Spanish text.

Having wolfed down a delicious, chunky and very garlicky paella, at junior-doctor speed, I gaze out into the crowds.

'Look! There's Liz over there. Just turning in front of the cathedral. See? *There*. With that man from reception – what's-'is-name. You know. They're holding hands. Did you see them? He's that very chatty one. Well, what-do-you-know?'

'I thought she was with the singer from the bar... erm, Lee.' Tom pauses, a very dead pink prawn hooked on the end of his fork.

'Maybe Liz knew Lee from a previous cruise – or maybe he's already been on board for months and they've got friendly.' Liz and her companion disappear from view.

'Mm,' says Tom, munching the prawn.

Back on board I approach the Medical Centre door to hear Coralie's voice: 'Bloody nurse too... cow... doing my head in...' The 'cow' must be me. Liz will have told Coralie that I've been a nurse. I step in and behave as though everything is normal.

'Hi. Who's on tonight?' I ask.

'I am,' says Liz.

'I'm off,' Coralie says, as she turns and promptly leaves. I might say, flounces off.

'Good day?' I ask Liz, trying to keep the air clear.

'Really good thanks,' she looks up, composing her face. 'I was escort on the tour to La Laguna.'

'Were you?' Hadn't I seen Liz in town with one of the reception staff? 'What was that like?' I stand awkwardly by the desk.

'It's a village about ten kilometres away – really pretty. The houses are painted different colours and the whole place is historic. Used to be the old capital apparently. The university's there too. We all had a meal in this old hall, like a community centre type of thing. Wine, a sort of meat stew, cheese, the whole business. Luckily there was nothing for me to do.' Liz gets notes out of the filing cabinet and unlocks the pharmacy door. I start to relax.

'Why? What might there be to do?'

'Don't you know about escorting? You're responsible for rounding up all the people on your tour. Tell a lie. There was an old man who got lost in a side street and I had to run and find him. Of course, there's always a local guide, but I have to count everyone there and back and see to people if they feel sick or fall over, you know – anything really. Carry spare loo rolls.' Liz sniggers. 'Listen. You should volunteer. You get a free trip. Ask at the tour desk.'

'Mm, sounds like a good idea. One of the dance hosts talked about it.' I move into my consulting room.

'I've seen you and your husband dancing in the Pool Bar. You're pretty good dancers, aren't you?' Liz looks round the door at me.

'Do you dance?' I ask.

'I did as a kid – ballet and tap, that sort of thing. The can-can. I remember holding my leg up straight in the air with my knee on my ear and hopping round on the other foot. Then we'd all leap up and land down in the splits. I was six. The teacher told Mum I'd be a good dancer if I practised, but I never practised. I haven't danced properly for ages now though. Just bopping in the crew discos.' Liz is standing holding a file in her hand.

'But did you see the carnival?' I ask, changing the subject. 'Loads of people in fancy dress. And big men dressed in drag. Weren't they just fascinating?'

'Yeah, when I got back from the tour. Seen it before. A bit weird if you ask me.' She purses her lips. I am surprised. What with a nurse's experience of meeting all manner of folk, I expect her to be super-liberal about people's harmless self-expression. Liz is clearly not a Londoner.

'It's because they get the chance once a year to be someone else, I suppose, and in fact the whole thing started hundreds of years ago. Any more gastros?' I hold my breath.

'One definite. One possible – a man in three-three-two had a couple of episodes, so he's confined until we see what happens. Still, there should be four releases tomorrow.'

I breathe out. 'I should think so too. Oh, by the way, do you know if the port agent collected the stool samples?'

'He should have. I e-mailed him yesterday.' Liz stops what she's doing.

'Ah, but when he came this morning, they weren't bagged up and no request forms. Coralie wasn't here and I was flat out, so I had to send him away. He said he'd come back if he had time.'

'Shit!' Liz disappears into the specimen room. She returns making a face. '*No.* Still there. *Bloody nuisance.* Now we'll have to get them off at Cape Verde. *That'll* be worse than useless. No decent lab facilities. I don't know if they can even *test* for noro.' She sits down heavily, her lips pressed together.

'We'll just have to get fresh samples. These will be too old by the time we get to Cape Verde. They'll be bug cemeteries in three days. At least if we can send ten we'll've done what was asked.' We gaze at each other, heads shaking.

Liz looks away.

———⚓———

In the Pool Bar Liz is sitting with Lee at a table right at the back of the room in shadow. Their heads are together in intimate conversation. Liz looks up. We raise eyebrows and nod.

'The captain!' Tom whispers, as the automatic doors to the deck open and Captain Strom strides in with his Chief Officer, Tallak. I've never seen them in the Pool Bar. I glance over at Liz and wonder if fraternising in her uniform with one of the entertainers is allowed in this military-style set-up. She appears unfazed. Captain Strom looks inscrutable and nods to Tom and me in passing. I guess they are on their rounds checking out the ship. Good thing too. You never know what might be happening.

Carrie sings *That Old Feeling*, a 1950s hit from Anita O'Day. A lovely, slow jive. I check that the captain has disappeared before Tom and I step onto the floor. I'd feel self-conscious doing our chassés, spins, fall-aways and stop-gos with the captain looking on, especially with me in uniform. There are only a handful of people in the bar. The dance hosts must be down in the Ocean Lounge, where the ship's orchestra plays at the end of the evening cabaret. A couple of women we don't recognise are installed on the long leather bench. On the table in front of them sit pink drinks with red and green cherries on cocktail sticks and oriental-style paper umbrellas unfurled at the tops of the glasses.

'They look exotic,' I say as we pass by.

'Don't worry, no alcohol, Doctor – it's "Cyclone Cup", all fruit juice and ice,' says one of them.

'Oh ye-es?'

'No... *honestly*,' they chorus.

Next thing, Carrie is singing *For All We Know* by the Carpenters. It is perfect for Dad's invention, the Why Dance: hold tight and barely move. I tell Tom about Coralie's insulting remark and her prompt departure when I walked into the Medical Centre. 'So, what are you going to do?' he asks.

'I'm going to leave it for the time being.' I watch Carrie and Dave, not wanting to talk over the top of their performance.

'What you have to do is write everything down, even retrospectively, with dates and times. In case things don't improve. Because at some point, maybe after a specific incident, you'll have to notify whoever has to be notified,' Tom says. The trade unionist is speaking. I wave my hand to indicate that he should lower his voice.

'Dr Wallis,' I say.

'Whenever I see her, she always seems to be in a bad mood, or in a huge rush, or both. What's she like – I mean, really?'

I pause. 'Brittle.' I feel a sense of shame that I can't get to grips with the situation. Trouble is, there are only two nurses. I can't suspend one pending a disciplinary enquiry like I would do in my Practice at home. I'm not her employer. Maybe I have to ask Dr Wallis's advice. It dents my professional pride, having to ask for help on my first cruise, especially considering I'm responsible for personnel in my Practice in Newham.

One more dance. Carrie sings *Sweet Dreams* by Annie Lennox.

It's late. We get up to go. I pick up my bleep. It has recorded a call, but I've missed it. I go to the nearest phone. 'We have a passenger threatening to throw himself overboard. Can you please come?' Oleg, the Hotel Manager, urges.

Oleg is sitting next to a man I don't know at the rear of a nearly empty bar. 'This is Mr Wilson.' Mr Wilson's face is puffy and red. He doesn't look up.

'What's been going on?'

'I don't *want* the doctor. *He* can't do anything.'

Oleg says, 'Let her just talk to you.'

'All becaush we had a row. My wife saysh she… saysh she… doesn't want to be with me anymore. She saysh she's… she's… going to leave me. I can't *live* without her-r… I'll die.' He breaks out into loud sobs, sniffing hard. I motion for Oleg to leave us.

Never try to reason with someone who's drunk. My best bet is to get him to talk it all out until he is too exhausted to remember his plan – if indeed he has a plan. 'I'll jump over the shide if she leaves me. I *will*.' He glares at me, jabbing the air and pointing towards the ocean. Threatening. Good. He's not depressed, but still at risk of an impetuous act, if he is sober enough to climb over the four-foot handrail.

'Tell me what happened.'

'Ohh – don't ask me… *nothing…*' He holds his head in his hands. 'Nothing.' He sniffs again. 'She said she was fed up. *Fed up…* I don't even know what it's about…' I bet he does. 'We've rowed before… we have… but not like this… She's never said she'd leave… *never…* never…' His voice trails off. He shakes his head. 'She'sh my life… my whole life.'

'You've had rows before?'

'Yesh – plenty… sure… who doesn't? I bet even you do… But we make up… we make up, somehow… always make up.'

'How?'

'*I don't know*. Too many questions… *questions.*' He raises his voice, starts to get up, but falls back into the chair. Good. He won't get over the handrail.

'Mr Wilson, I'm trying to help. See if we can sort it out. Where is your wife now?'

'I *don't know*. In the cabin… but she won't speak to me. I love her. She knows I love her. I can't live without her… I *can't…*' He cries, wiping his eyes on his sleeve. He is becoming tired. 'Will *you* speak to her, Doc?'

'Sure.' Did I have a certificate in marriage guidance counselling? Did I heck. 'Why don't you find her and ask her to come up here. I'll be here for the next fifteen minutes. Or I can see her in surgery tomorrow. Yes?'

'I'll find her… and… and I'll bring her.' He leans his head forward towards his knees to gain sufficient momentum to get out of the chair.

'Excellent idea. I'll wait here for fifteen minutes. OK?'

'Mm.' He holds on to the furniture on his way out, staggering with a wide gait.

Fifteen minutes later I walk downstairs to the cabin.

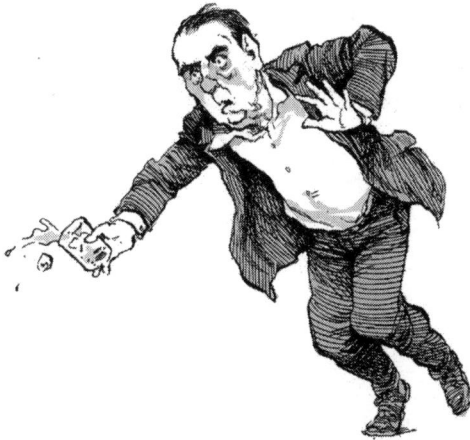

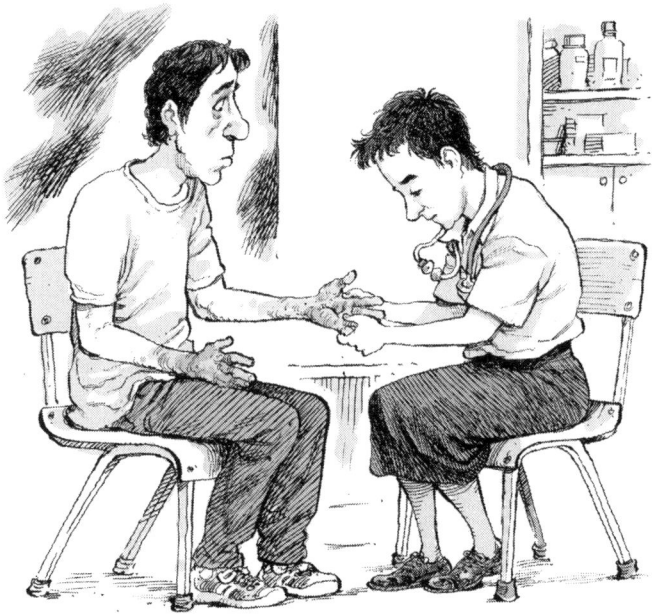

Day 8

Jesus

Every pot and pan, plate and dish, knife, fork and glass is washed by hand. No automatic dishwashers, just ten human handwashers in the galley. These kitchen hands join the ship as the lowest ratings. If they do their jobs well and get on with their work colleagues, they can earn promotion to peeling potatoes or cutting up vegetables for their next contract. Jesus has been a washer for four months of his eight-month stint.

'Look, my hands – very bad,' he says, holding out two pink, scaly extremities. 'I can't do my job no more.'

'Let me see.' I hold out my hands for him to put his in mine.

Red to the wrists, his skin looks angry, dry and scratched as though by a cat.

It is acute contact dermatitis from washing-up liquid. An allergy.

'Can you wear gloves – rubber gloves?' I am still holding his hands.

'I wear dem, but water comes over de top, inside de gloves.' He withdraws his hands, looking at them and rubbing them on his trousers.

'How long are your gloves?'

'To here.' Jesus indicates a level one third of the way up his forearm.

'Can't you get longer gloves?'

'I ask Chef but he say no.' His mouth turns down at the corners.

'OK. I'll speak to him. In the meantime, I want you to wash your hands in a special moisturising cream I'll give you. Don't use soap. And put ointment on after drying. Try to keep your hands dry when you're washing up, and I'll speak to Chef about longer gloves. OK? Come and see me in a week.'

Medical services are free for the crew. The nurses see crew members first to triage them, to decide if they need to see the doctor or whether they can manage the patients themselves. Crew can attend with minor illnesses such as a cough, cold, sore throat or sea-sickness, sometimes on the very morning that it starts. The nurses are authorised to dispense paracetamol and sea-sick pills or injections. The crews' contracts do not include a day off for eight months, yet many want to avoid a reputation for accruing sick leave, which might be held against them when signing on for the next contract. On the other hand, if they can legitimately be signed off sick for a day or two, some welcome the brief period of complete respite. For me, their sick leave presents a management and an ethical dilemma.

Liz has reviewed the noros first thing.

'Four discharged,' she announces triumphantly. 'And the observation man from yesterday has had nothing since, so he can be discharged this afternoon. He's not a case.'

'Great! At least the numbers are coming down... give me some of those to ring.'

Liz hands me a wadge of notes. The phone rings. Two new cases. A husband and wife.

'Uh-oh. I've jinxed it. I'll shut up. But we can get a couple of stool samples. What's the stool score?'

'Only one. I've chucked the rest. Listen. We'll have to collect some before Cape Verde, though honestly, we're wasting our time. I don't remember them *ever* testing for noro. They have to send the samples away to God-knows-where. They're hundreds of miles from anywhere. It's practically the third world.' Liz purses her lips.

Ruby Wilson comes in for a blood pressure check.

'How are those headaches?' Suddenly it starts to dawn. Is Ruby the wife of Mr Wilson of throwing-himself-overboard fame? Funny, I really can't visualise them as a couple.

'A bit better, I think. Not quite gone though. It's right at the front – here.' She pinches her forehead hard between finger and thumb and grimaces.

'Right, your blood pressure's... one hundred and seventy over... ninety-five. So that's better than it was, but needs to come down even more. Can you do a urine sample?' I hand her a container. 'And how have you got on with your eating?'

'I've tried to be good, Doctor, honestly, but it's really hard. There are so many nice things which I don't make at home. And it's all just sitting in front of you on the buffet asking to be picked up.' She gives a wry smile.

It is always a difficult balance trying to encourage the patient to limit their food intake, while avoiding making them feel so bad about themselves that they comfort-eat.

I write up her notes while Liz checks her blood sugar and urine.

Mrs Wilson sits down and sighs.

'Your sugar is eight point eight – acceptable – and your urine is fine, so your kidneys seem to be OK, which is good. Have you had any stresses on board that might have contributed to the headaches?'

'Well, as you've asked – I suppose I have. It's my husband. He drinks too much, more than ever on board. I've put up with it for years but I don't know how much longer I can stand it. It's getting me down something awful. We've been having rows – really bad arguments. The next-door cabins must hear us. I don't know if I even want to be with him anymore. What can you do for alcoholics? He *is* an alcoholic. He gets so nasty when he drinks. I don't know what to do. My children won't have anything to do with him. They're from my first marriage. I don't see them. They can't stand him… Oh, I don't know, Doctor…'

'Do you want to see me together?'

'He's so stubborn. I'll ask him, but I don't expect he'll come.'

'I'll need to check you in three days. Bring Mr Wilson then if he'll come, or sooner if you can.'

I bleep the Head Chef, Lenz. 'I've seen one of your galley-hands today, name of Jesus. He has a bad case of detergent dermatitis. He says water comes over the top of his gloves. Have you got any longer gloves?'

'The company doesn't supply long gloves. He has standard issue. He already complained to me about it. None of the others have this problem. He's careless. Don't put him off sick. I need all my washers.' Lenz sounds harassed.

'Is there anything you *can* do? His hands *are* bad.'

'OK. I can take him

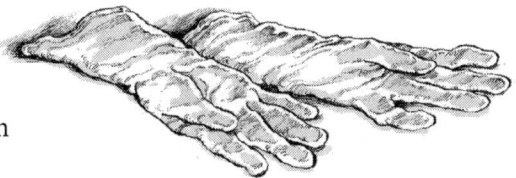

off the sinks for a few days, maybe two or three, but then he'll have to go back on. That's just it. He doesn't want to wash up. He wants to be moved.'

'Is there any chance of him being moved?'

'No. Not him. Wrong attitude.' Chef's voice becomes hard.

'What do you mean "wrong attitude"?'

'Resentful.'

'Well, look, any time off the sinks would be helpful. Is there someone I can speak to about the gloves? I mean, who orders them?'

'Quartermaster. Gary Pearce. Speak to Gary.'

I ring.

'Who wants me?' He has a matter-of-fact Cockney accent.

'It's the doctor. Gary, I have a galley-man with hand dermatitis. His washing-up gloves aren't long enough. Water comes over the top. Do you have longer ones?'

'No, they're the regular size. We don't keep long gloves.' There is resistance in his voice.

'Can you order some?'

'Just for one crewman? No, I can't order for one person.'

'Well, what if all the washer-uppers were given them?' Industrial relations.

'That'd 'ave to come from Head Office. 'E'll 'ave to go ashore and buy a couple of pairs 'imself, if 'e can find 'em.'

I feel defeated. I wonder whether Gary would order something special if the patient was an officer occupying the top deck as opposed to a seaman from below decks.

In the afternoon I phone Mr Armsure.

'How are you this evening?' I ask, visualising him in his striped pyjamas.

'I'm champion, Doc. But I tell yer, I'd feel a lot better if I could get some fresh air.'

'No more symptoms?'

'Nowt while yesterday. Can't I get out now?'

I can hear Harold shouting, 'Yes, yer *did*. *Tell the doctor*. You went this morning.'

Albert shouts, '*No*, but that were just *ord'nary*. It weren't liquid, it were more soft-like.'

''appen, but the doctor *wants to know*.'

'I'm *tellin'* 'er!'

I look at his record.

'You can't go quite yet, Mr Armsure. It'll be the day after tomorrow. It has to be forty-eight hours after your last symptom because the bug hangs around in your body for a few days after you're better and you'll be shedding it in the toilet. We have to allow time for it to get out of your system. All being well, you and Harold will be discharged just in time for Cape Verde in two days. Don't leave the cabin until we give you the all-clear.'

'That'll be grand. I'll be that 'appy to get some fresh air. Air's right stale in 'ere. It keeps going round 'n' round.'

'Actually,' I put in, 'fresh sea air is being drawn in continuously from the outside through your air-conditioning. It doesn't get recirculated.'

'Are you su-re?'

'Yes, that's straight from the Chief Engineer, from the horse's mouth.'

'Ee. I didn't know that. I'll tell 'arold.'

⚓

I hold the telephone in both hands, weighing it, looking at it. I take one hand off. Then dial.

I tell Dr Wallis the whole Coralie saga. He listens.

'Leave it with me. I'll see to it.'

—⚓—

That afternoon Reg attends. It feels like I'm treating an uncle who has boundary issues. Can I be objective knowing Reg socially? In Newham I made a point of not socialising with my patients, wanting to maintain a professional distance. It didn't really work. Some patients I liked better than others, so I found myself treating my 'special patients' more favourably. The 'professional distance' shortened.

'It's this rash,' Reg says. 'It started on my stomach, now it's all over. So itchy. I'm waking up scratching in the night. What is it?'

I ask Reg to expose his abdomen. It looks unusual. There are showers of tiny, flat, red spots; I mean really miniscule – some areas look like he's sucked blood into the skin the way we did as children on our forearms. Most are on his chest and stomach. I avoid asking him to show me where they've spread below the waist.

I want to write GOK in his notes – God Only Knows.

But after asking about skincare products, I diagnose an allergy to the ship's shower gel, so prescribe an unperfumed cream wash and antihistamines. No charge.

—⚓—

After dinner I sign the Port Health Declaration for Cape Verde. It's now a stable routine. Done.

In the Pool Bar, Tom is on the sofa in conversation with two women. I join him.

His older sofa companion has a small pretty face, made up with eyeliner and pale blue eyeshadow, all framed by bright, white, well-coiffed short hair. The younger one has high cheekbones and bright red lipstick. Her eyes dart about, taking in everything, and sparkle when they fix on a face. Four dance hosts stroll in, smart in white trousers and blue blazers, nod greetings to the four of us and sit down nearby.

Tom and I move tables, out of earshot, to catch up with each other's news and to gossip, talking about everything and nothing.

'Do you know those women?' I ask.

'No, I'm innocent! I was sitting on my own and Pat comes up to me and says, "You look shy. Are you by yourself? Come and sit with us." I say, "No, I'm not on my own, I'm the doctor's husband. She's on duty. And actually, I'm one of the least shy people you could meet." She said, "Have you been married long?" I said, "No. What about you? Have you got a partner?" She said, "No. All the men I get don't stay. I want someone permanent." I didn't know if it was an invitation or a cry for help. Alice, the older one, she's a widow. She's from Wigan. Her husband and her used to do a lot of ballroom dancing – medals, cups and all that stuff that you've got. Competitions as well. Blackpool Tower for all I know. She's working class. Apparently, she's got a heart condition. But you wouldn't know to look at her,' he confides, although gossip never seems to be confidential to Tom. It's just public information.

'What sort of a heart condition?' Now I am curious.

'*I* don't *know*. I didn't ask her.'

'She looks well enough,' I say, glancing across at her slim ankles. No fluid retention there.

Lee is playing. Liz is nowhere to be seen. He starts singing *Let's Get Lost*, a favourite of his. A quickstep.

'This is *so* old-fashioned. It must be 1940s. Why can't he play something modern?' Tom opines.

'He's playing it just for you. It's from your youth.'

'You *had* to say that, didn't you?' We chuckle.

The dance hosts are up on the floor with their charges. Alice is doing a feather-light quickstep with all the advanced moves Peter can throw in. They look a well-matched couple, both petite, moving effortlessly with their neat elaborate footwork. In their element. Alice isn't even breathless.

Brian, over six feet, with an unwieldy mop of curly grey hair and big feet, is dancing with Pat. They both manage a fair quickstep, stopping to laugh as they tread on each other's toes.

'*Come on*, let's do the quickstep.' I am dying to get on the floor.

'Oh, no-o.' Tom looks pained. 'Let's see what the next one is. I'll do whatever the next one is.' His face says: *I-will-not-be-moved*.

'What about the port talk?'

'This is interesting – apparently Cape Verde was a coaling station for steam ships crossing the Atlantic, and a slave distribution port for the Portuguese slave trade. Apart from that, he made it sound as though there's nothing there.'

The coffee is undrinkable on board what with its desalinated sea water and UHT milk. It is a pleasure to plan our next two-hour holiday. Tom is to run round the port and find the number one coffee spot.

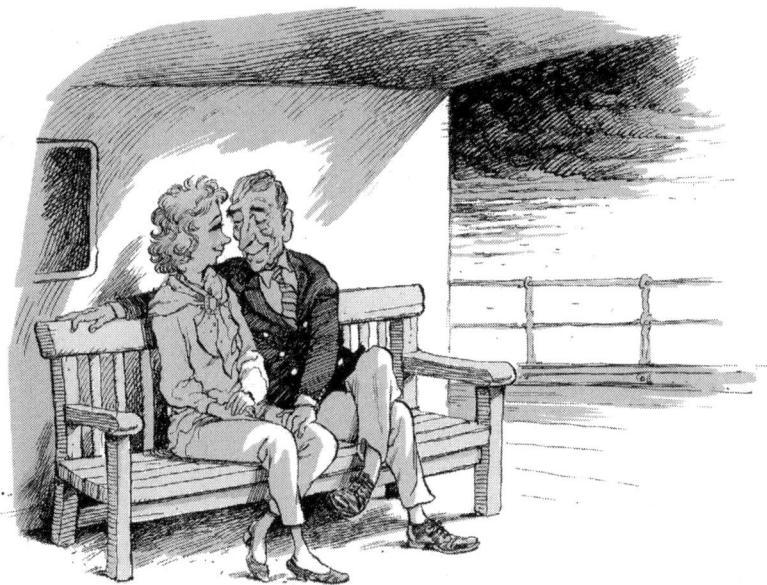

Day 9

Mr Richardson

The day starts with no nurse. I ring Coralie.

'Ye-ess.'

'Coralie, are you meant to be on duty?' A hard edge to my voice.

'Yeah – ohh Christ!'

'How long will you be?' I am not sympathetic.

'Dunno. Twenty minutes?'

'Quick as you can.' It is as near to an order as I can muster.

The phone goes dead. There is nothing else for it. WORDS will have to be spoken – again.

I start ringing the gastros. My calls can't be shorter. There are no new gastros in the log and we are at last discharging more than we are confining.

Coralie walks in. Her face looks swollen. She neither greets me, nor apologises, nor looks me in the eye. I breathe out heavy with aggravation like the steam that used to hiss out of Mum's pressure cooker.

Eleanor, the engineer shop-steward we met in the Pool Bar, attends with cystitis. The urine dipstick shows signs of infection. I give her antibiotics. I wonder if it is 'honeymoon cystitis' as a result of her close encounters with the dance host, Edward. Not so much a waltz as a tango. If so, would she have also caught a sexually transmitted infection?

'Anything else?' A question I ask like the proverbial barber's 'Anything for the weekend, sir?'

'No. That's it, thanks,' Eleanor says. I believe her.

I hope she knows that everything is confidential in the consulting room, as opposed to the Chinese whispers that regularly roll around the ship like sea mist.

Voices are raised outside.

'I'll have my money back!'

'You can't have your money back… you've had the services.' It's Coralie's voice.

'Call it a service! I'm no better and you've kept charging me for useless treatment! It's daylight robbery!' It's Mr Wayfield.

My first thought is to escape back through the thin ward door into my cabin and hide under the bed. But I leave the office and walk towards the commotion like a fire-fighter towards the fire. Mr Wayfield is facing Coralie in the waiting area, red-faced, wild-eyed and gesticulating. *'It's a bloody swindle.'*

'Come in, Mr Wayfield. Come in.' I don't want this ruction in the waiting room, with other patients observing the shenanigans.

We stand in the office, face to face. It is a duel.

'Your antibiotics are a load of rubbish! Not done a thing! Not a blind bit of good. I'm *not* paying for them! Here, you can have them back! And I'll have my money back too!'

He throws the antibiotic packet down on the desk. They land with a thwack.

'I can't give your money back, Mr Wayfield. You've already had three consultations, and you've had medication.'

'Fat lot of good it's done me! *Useless.* I'm no better. In fact, I'm *worse!* Why should I pay for useless treatment? I'm entitled to a refund!' His eyes are popping, his body rigid.

I am in a losing position. And worse still, patients in the waiting area can still overhear the furious accusations.

'Come with me for a minute. Come in. Come in. Let's see if we can sort this out.' I motion for him to follow me into the consulting room.

'I'm not paying a penny more! I'm telling you now!' He glares as he leans against my desk.

'OK,' I say, not knowing whether there is a legitimate route to a refund.

'Now start from the beginning,' I say, waving him into the chair.

'Well, *you* know as well as *I* do. This cough won't *shift.* The wife and I can't *sleep.* I've told you before. You're not *listening.* I *daren't* go to our dining table. We've been eating in the *buffet* restaurant for three days.'

'Yes, I can see that the cough is very persistent.'

'*Persistent?* It's *this boat.* It's the *air-conditioning. That's* what's the problem. The *same* air's being circulated *round and round,* spreading the germs. It's bad air. Tons of people have got this cough. I've *heard* them all round the ship.'

'Actually, you know, the air-conditioning draws fresh sea air into the ship continuously. It doesn't circulate,' I say, thinking this will be a clincher.

'Well, *you* explain it then, if you're so clever. Why am I still coughing? You tell *me.*' He leans towards me. I can feel his breath on my face.

'Your breathing tubes are obviously very irritated. I think it calls for a proper inhalation treatment. I'd like you to try it. No charge. Will you do that for me?'

'That's all very well, but what about all those other charges?' Maybe he thinks I make up the charges and pay myself the proceeds.

'Leave it with me, Mr Wayfield. I'll see to it… Coralie?' I call out, opening the door. 'Can you set up a saline inhalation for Mr Wayfield via the nebuliser,' I lower my voice, 'with added TLC.' I hope he doesn't hear, but if he does, he'll imagine there is some powerful extra medication added. (TLC – Tender Loving Care.)

Coralie wordlessly goes into the treatment room.

I usher Mr Wayfield after Coralie and with relief leave them to it. 'Nurse Coralie will see to everything,' I say, hoping that at least she won't be bad-tempered with *him*. A minute later I can hear her fussing round him.

When I go in Mr Wayfield is sitting in the treatment room, surrounded by emergency equipment, with a mask strapped to his face delivering the inhalation, the nebuliser puttering like a big purring cat. He looks like a proper patient, serious and suffering.

'Are you OK?' asks Dr Concerned.

'Mmm,' he murmurs, unaware that he can speak with the mask on.

'Very good. Just breathe normally. You don't have to take deep breaths,' I say, looking at him for longer than I need to, increasing the Dose of Doctor, and resting my hand on his shoulder. 'Stay put until nurse or I have checked you over.'

The office phone rings.

'We've been kept in our cabin for four days. *Four days*. We only came on the trip to go to the carnival and now we've missed it. We're entitled to compensation. We've missed four whole days of a very expensive cruise.'

I look at the gastro log.

'You were released yesterday, weren't you?'

'Yes. That's all very well, but we've missed the most important port. There must be reimbursement. How do we claim? Do you have to write us a letter?'

I confirm the cabin number. It is Mr Royston, whose wife had wanted champagne and canapés in the cabin on the first Formal Night. Being on an upper deck, they will have paid a great deal for their cruise. Thousands, possibly tens of thousands. The higher up the ship, the bigger the cabins, including a sitting room and private balcony.

Surely the company won't give compensation to all these gastro passengers. It's not the company's fault. I agree to find out.

I go back to Mr Wayfield. 'All well?' asks Dr-Caring-and-Sympathetic.

'Yes.' He realises he can speak now.

'Are you feeling any better?' I venture.

'Mmm. A bit.'

'Good. It often does help.' I hype up the optimism.

Coralie comes in. A Double Dose of Medical Personnel.

'Keep checking Mr Wayfield until this is finished, please Coralie, then if he's OK, we can let him go. No charge. And I suggest another inhalation this evening. Would that be alright with you, Mr Wayfield? Can you come back this evening?' says Dr Creepily-Wheedling.

'Yes. Alright. What time?' His eyes flick up to mine.

'Just come down anytime. See you this evening then,' I say. I leave Coralie with him and can overhear them in therapeutic conversation.

After surgery I call Coralie into the consulting room.

'Are you having trouble getting up in the mornings?'

'Yeah – alarm clock's not working,' she says, glancing at me, using her fringe as a refuge.

'It makes it very difficult for me if I'm on my own down here, you know. Can you get reception to give you a morning call? Or get a new alarm clock?' The last question is more confrontational than sympathetic.

'I expect so.' She isn't going to engage.

'When's your next morning on?'

'I dunno… err… thirteenth.'

'Can you be in on time on the thirteenth then?'

'I'll try.'

'Right. That'd be very helpful,' I say, as though it is all cordially agreed.

***

After dinner Tom and I decide to take a turn around the deck. The air is warm and salty on our faces. Over the rail, swishing white foam tumbles by, while further out deep blackness takes over in a void to infinity. The sea has been put to bed.

'Coralie didn't come in again this morning – until I rang her in her cabin. She was *asleep*. I had to have Words.'

'You're putting me on! You've given her a second warning?' We walk along arm in arm.

'I don't know what you'd call it. But I can't put up with this – on my own in surgery, filling out paperwork, answering the phone, seeing patients, sorting out medication. Not to mention the billing. *Too much.* I rang Dr Wallis yesterday. He says he'll see to it. I've left it with him. And guess what? A passenger came in wanting his money back because I hadn't made him better. Imagine!'

'He did *not*!'

'I gave him free treatment. It reminds me of the old Chinese system where the patient paid the doctor if they got better and the doctor paid the patient if they didn't. A pretty good system,

I'd say. It'd put charlatans and bad doctors out of business, that's for sure. Trouble is, it would encourage hypochondriacs never to get better, and the NHS would go bankrupt.'

We pass another couple strolling in the opposite direction, and exchange evening greetings.

'Anyway, I've organised free inhalations for him twice a day. It gives him a high dose of nurse and doctor, so that should work.'

'You know where I sit up on deck eight, at those tables? Well, a woman came up to me while I was drawing and said, "Aren't you the doctor's husband?" I said, "Yes, but I'm not medical." She took no notice and said, "I don't want to bother her. I know how busy she is, but could you just ask her if she's got any of these pills," and she showed me a handful of little blue pills. Really small. Tiny. Of course, I didn't have a clue what they were and I...'

Just then a passenger walks up to us from behind and stands by my side. 'Doctor, excuse me. I just want to ask you if you think my tablets could be making my legs swell.' She lifts her dress and sticks her leg out. 'They're for blood pressure – oh, and I take one for cholesterol.'

Her leg doesn't look swollen to me. 'Well, they could, but really I'd need to see you properly in surgery with your medication.' I give her my this-is-the-end-of-the-consultation nod. We try ambling on. She keeps up with us.

'I thought I'd just ask. I don't want to trouble you in surgery. I know you're very busy. Do you think I can just stop them and see if my legs go down?'

'No. I wouldn't do that – especially blood pressure pills. Come down and see me in the Medical Centre and bring all your tablets, then we can sort it out properly. No need to book.'

'I see. Thanks doctor, I knew you wouldn't mind...'

These 'corridor consultations' are downright dangerous. No

proper history, no examination, lots of details missing and no record kept. I juggle feelings of frustration at never being off duty, at Tom and I having our perambulation interrupted, and at the thought that passengers who are used to the NHS probably want to avoid paying fees. At the same time, I do not want to be deliberately off-putting or alternatively seen as touting for business.

Around the bow the wind is fierce as the ship heads into it at sixteen knots. I lean against the current of air, realising now why I couldn't have worn the tricorn hat. There is no good light at the front but we can just make out a necking couple on a bench situated in the gloom under the overhang of the Bridge. It looks like Reginald grappling with a younger woman. He has his hand on her bare thigh. The couple are pressed together, clothes and hair flapping in the gale, kissing passionately.

As we make our way towards the Pool Bar, Tom exclaims, 'Did you see that? It *was* Reg, wasn't it? What do you make of that? Clearly there's a bit of life in the old dog yet.'

'It *was* Reg. I can't believe it. But who's *she*? I didn't recognise her.'

'Looked a bit like Barbara to me.'

'Who's Barbara?'

'You know. One of the women who goes to the Pool Bar. Sits with Pat and the dance hosts and that lot.'

'But would you *credit* it? I mean, Reg? *Honestly.*'

'What a lad! You just never know… I'll point Barbara out to you next time I see her,' says Tom.

Suddenly, *The Great Imitator* comes to mind. In student lectures in the '70s we'd been taught over and again that syphilis imitates many other conditions, especially the syphilitic rash. Could this have been what caused Reg's rash, considering the Barbara factor?

My bleep sounds. A passenger has fallen out of bed.

'Sorry. Have to go. I'll be back,' I tell Tom, hurrying off to his familiar look of abandonment.

Coralie is in the patient's cabin, getting him into a wheelchair. He is conscious and cooperating. 'This is Mr Richardson,' Coralie says, tucking his dressing gown in around his knees.

His wife says, 'John never falls out of bed. But he didn't feel at all well today. He went to bed early. It's not like him.'

'Are you on any tablets, Mr Richardson?' I ask.

'Yes,' he pants, 'in the drawer.' He waves his hand vaguely towards the dressing table and closes his eyes.

'He's diabetic,' says his wife.

'Can you bring along all his medication, Mrs Richardson?' I say, 'and we'll take you down to the Medical Centre to check you out, sir.' Coralie is already wheeling him out.

Once in the hospital, Mrs Richardson recounts that her husband has been coughing for over a week, worse in the previous forty-eight hours. He's become breathless doing normal things and is now refusing food. Mr Richardson appears too exhausted to talk.

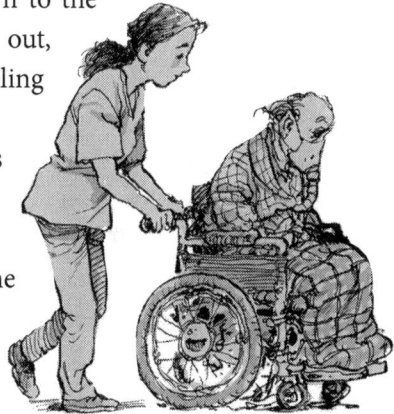

His examination reveals a high fever of 40.2°C, a racing heart, and abnormal sounds in his chest.

Coralie does his ECG, which apart from the fast heartbeat looks pretty normal. His blood sugar is 14.7mmol/L – a little high for a type two diabetic but not high enough to start insulin. Coralie tests his urine for ketones (a sign of diabetes being out of control) and infection. The results are clear. His blood oxygen level is lower than I would like, but then he is seventy-eight and ill.

I bring my face closer to his. 'Mr Richardson. It looks like you've got a chest infection.'

'See, I said you weren't well. I told you to go to the doctor's but you wouldn't go, would you?' Mrs Richardson chides, pursing her lips.

'Well, good thing you're here now,' I say. 'You'll need antibiotics. Are you allergic to anything?'

'There was one that upset my stomach. Vera, what was it?'

'Ohh… I can't remember,' says Vera, drawing in her breath. 'Was that the one for your leg?'

'I don't know. Did it start with L?… Or was it flossy-something?'

'Never mind,' I say, 'we wouldn't normally class a stomach upset as an allergy. It's usually an itchy rash or face swelling. But I can't be sure that there isn't a slight pneumonia in there.' I like the word 'slight' – less frightening than plain, out-with-it 'pneumonia'. 'So I'll arrange for you to have a chest X-ray in Mindelo tomorrow.'

'Alright.' Mr Richardson closes his eyes again, and drops his head forward. He looks as though he will agree to anything. Arguing is usually a sign of rude health.

Coralie dispenses antibiotics and paracetamol, helps Mrs Richardson to sign the insurance forms, then wheels him back up to his cabin.

Fifteen minutes later Coralie returns. 'Thanks for doing all that,' I say. 'How do I organise his X-ray for tomorrow?'

She switches on the computer. 'Here are the port agents. Mindelo's is in there.' She points to a file on the desktop. 'Send him an e-mail. He'll arrange it, and then you copy to all this lot.' She hands me a protocol manual and opens it at the 'Referrals' page. 'Do a letter to the hospital. Oh, and e-mail the insurance company. Here. You'll have to fill out the medical details on the insurance forms and get reception to fax them.' She tidies up, says, 'OK. I'm off,' and leaves.

I e-mail the port agent about the chest X-ray and transport. Copies go to Dr Wallis, the Nurses, the Captain, the Chief Officer, the Security Officer, the Reception Manager, Hotel Manager, the Housekeeping Manager, the Maître d', and Customer Relations. Uncle Tom Cobley and all. So much for patient confidentiality. I complete the medical report to the hospital, followed by an e-mail to the insurance company. Over an hour and a half has passed.

I switch off the lights and shut the door. The phone rings. I go back in. It is Mr Richardson's insurance company. 'Dr Taylor, we need a copy of your letter to the hospital. Could you e-mail it to us now?' *Now*? I hit the light switch, slap open the computer and bang out the e-mail, swearing at my typos.

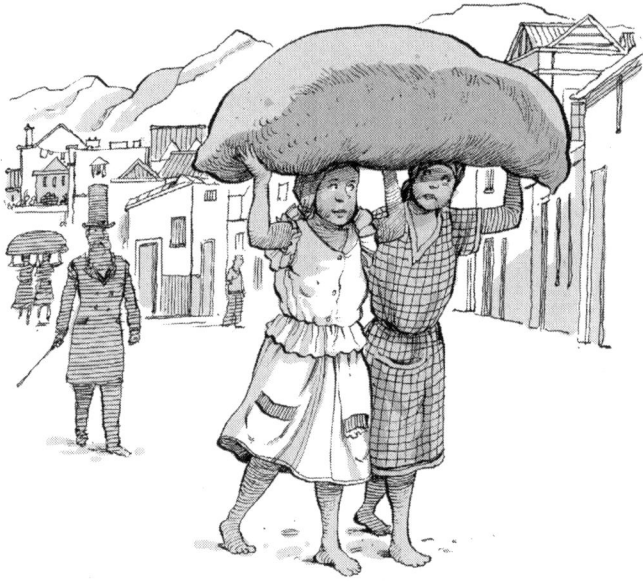

Day 10

Rosa

We dock in the deep harbour of Mindelo, on the Cape Verde island of Sao Vicente. I lean over the handrail. The quay is basalt black, spattered with bright yellow spots. Local men are loading a battered open-backed lorry high with unwanted goods from the ship. Deck-hands are passing broken chairs and tables, lengths of old carpet, fire extinguishers, discarded catering equipment and linen from a short platform low down on the ship's side to the three men on the back of the truck. I rouse myself, suddenly aware that Coralie might be absent again, and run down to the Medical Centre.

Mr Wayfield is standing, waiting. I smile and nod to him, providing a preliminary Dose of Doctor; a homeopathic dose, but containing a memory of the full strength.

It's a relief to see Liz already in, putting down the phone from a gastro call.

I lower my voice. 'Mr Wayfield's outside – you know, the man whose cough won't go. He's having saline inhalations via the nebuliser, and lots of TLC. Could you take him into the treatment room when you're ready?'

'How many times a day?' Liz calls out from the treatment room. At least her behaviour towards me is normal.

'Twice.' I go in, not wanting to shout the conversation. 'But as often as he wants, if you're free. Oh, and no charge. I can do that, can't I? Is it me who decides whether passengers pay or not?' Liz looks up.

'Well, the company has its scale of charges. You know all about them, but *you* can decide. You know the gastros aren't charged for *anything* related to gastro, but *you* still get a fee if you telephone them or do a cabin visit.'

'I didn't know that. Shouldn't I be keeping a record?'

'No, we've got all the records here. They go up to Lisa in Accounts at the end of your contract.'

'So, no charge for Mr Wayfield, and can you cancel the cost of his last consultation and the antibiotics?'

'Sure.'

'I'll see him after the inhalation. Now, Mr Richardson in three-one-nine is going ashore for a chest X-ray. Possible pneumonia. His stuff is on the desk. When the port agent rings will you let the Richardsons know the arrangements?'

An e-mail from the Sanitation Officer informs me that I have Sanitation Training at eleven a.m. Damn. I ring Tom. 'I wondered what'd happened to you,' he says, as if I'd jumped ship.

'Sorry, I got caught up with a patient.' The number of times he's heard that since we've been together – countless. Always late home from surgery or returning from a home visit that has taken twice as long as anticipated.

I ring Mr Armsure. 'Any more symptoms?'

'No. Nowt. To tell the truth, I'm a bit t'other way – you know, 'ard to go.'

In the background Harold calls out, 'Doctor doesn't want to know about *that*.'

'Well, once you're out and about I expect that'll right itself,' I say.

'Ee, I can't wait while I get on t' dry land.'

'Ask her about *drinking water* in t' port,' Harold shouts.

'Oh yes. What can I drink when I'm out, doctor?'

'Anything bottled, or boiled – like tea, but no ice if it's a cold drink. I have to move on now, Mr Armsure. You enjoy Cape Verde.'

⚓

Mr Wayfield finishes his inhalation.

'How's the chest feeling?' My hand is on his arm as I look down at him.

'A bit easier. I'm coughing less. Why didn't I have this from the start?' he says, staring up at me. I let go of his arm.

'It's always difficult to know what will work in any one person. Everyone is such an individual.' I left it at that. Basically, it was a case of S.M. – Search Me. 'I've cancelled your last bill. Is that OK?'

'OK,' is all he says, standing up.

'You can have the inhalations for as long as they're helpful. I suspect the cough will gradually dwindle and disappear now.' I'm dispensing the Doctor as Medicine – not quite placebo but acknowledging the patient's suffering and encouraging him in the recovery process. In the background Liz is doing gastro discharges. For the first time there are no new cases.

⚓

The same windowless lower deck mess room is host to Sanitation Training. The motley collection of crew from assorted departments lounge on the seats at the back, some chatting, a couple dozing.

As far as my concentration allows, there is much talk about white water, which is clean uncontaminated water, and grey water, from showers and baths, being discharged into the ocean. The coyly named black water, or sewage, is apparently treated in a huge septic tank of some sort, filtered and discharged into the sea as liquid when the bacteria have been neutralised – like the process in sewage farms at home. I don't like the idea of the environmental impact, making a mental note to look up the evidence when I get back. Bilge water, a mixture of oil and water, is discharged to a port container.

Mario, the Sanitation Officer, is a diminutive man with a strong Filipino accent, and a mop of black hair that stands up in insolent spikes on the crown of his head. His youthful face belies ten years of experience in shipping sanitation. Using a white baton he taps the PowerPoint presentation, simultaneously clicking his tongue, stating, 'Paper put in ve green bag, bottles and cans in ve red bag, ubber waste in ve black bag. You see vem in ve crew mess. Don't mix vem up. Ve sanitation crew have to separate eberyving.' He talks about the water testing of the pools, jacuzzis and shower heads – 'for coliform and legionella', the common noxious microbes that can cause havoc on board. At last Mario says, 'Collect your certificate before you leave.' Another certificate.

Back in the cabin I am changing into an orange sun dress and sandals when Tom bursts in, panting, in a sweat-stained t-shirt, shorts and trainers.

'Phew! The roads are *terrible...* you won't believe it... they're made out of great blocks of rock – with these huge gaps between them. I nearly twisted my ankle twice. I could have easily fallen over. And the place is *so poor*. So undeveloped. I bet you they're sorry they became independent from Portugal now that Portugal's part of the EU. They could do with a bit of EU funding right now. Which makes the *massive* villas on the outskirts of town so *obscene*. They all seem to be surrounded by wire fences, patrolled by vicious-looking Alsatians. I bet you they belong to ex-pats who've made money abroad. But the rest's *terribly* poor. *You'll* see. The ordinary people have *nothing*. Oh... and... nothing's open either. No cafés or coffee shops. You'd think they'd welcome the tourist trade – at *least* open the shops while the ship's in. I just can't understand it. Forget Sunday. If I was a shopkeeper I'd make sure I opened when a ship arrived and stayed open till it left. There can't be that much chance of making money here. I mean – what *is* their source of income?' Tom disappears into the bathroom.

'Ex-pat Cape Verdeans abroad and foreign aid, I seem to remember from the guidebook. Here we are – the ship's map shows a tourist office in the port – we could ask about a café there,' I call out.

'I saw it. I tell you, it's really just a tiny hut. *Tiny*. Nothing,' he shouts back.

'Still, they'd know what's open.' Determined to make my point. Last wordism.

After lunch we step ashore into the shimmering heat. A blanket of fine dust hangs in the air like a thin veil. On the dockside the yellow spots I'd seen from the ship turn out to be corn kernels spilled across the black volcanic slabs, presumably during loading or unloading of maize. The brown mountains of Sao Vicente fold their distant peaks around Mindelo's bay.

It reminds me of Anselm Kiefer's sculpture containing corn to represent the loss of the seed corn of Jewish lives in the Holocaust. The artwork consisted of a massive black, lead-leaved open book within a monumental lead library, big enough to walk into, the books imprisoning the corn kernels in their pages.

I think of the seed corn of black slaves' lives sacrificed during the four centuries when Portuguese colonists used these uninhabited islands to process slaves from the West African coast for export to the Americas. No cruise-ship luxury for them. From Cape Verde they were transported in chains in the leaking wooden sailing ships of the day, some going down in storms on the way, sick slaves being thrown overboard. Cape Verde ended up with ten times more Africans living there than Portuguese by the time slavery was abolished in 1833. We are cruising the slave trade route.

In the centre of Mindelo is a street market; in fact, more of a pavement sale. 'Tom. Look there. All that stuff for sale. That's all the bric-a-brac from the ship. I saw it being loaded onto a truck on the dockside.'

Two men are sitting on broken chairs on the pavement, overseeing transactions. A group of locals mill around the wares, turning them over and bargaining with the sellers, pointing out the defects and gesticulating.

'If the locals are lucky, the shipping company pays for them to take it all away, and clearly it's a bit of an earner for the men if they can sell it on. Good. And *there's* the tourist kiosk. See? I told you. It's not worth bothering about.'

'Let's ask what's open at least. And they have postcards too, by the door. Look! Good-o.' I am already excited about being in a new place, foreign, colourful, and not Newham. I want to send a postcard to Dad telling him about the trip.

The tourist office looks like one of those sweet-and-crisp-booths on the platform of a British railway station, just big enough for one person to stand in. A woman in her thirties, hair braided into a dozen narrow woven plaits, wearing a bright yellow blouse, faces us with an apathetic expression. She turns our ship-issued map round several times and mutters something in her language, then pushes it away and opens her own map.

'Here is Mindel Hotel,' she says. 'Is a bar on top. You have drinks and coffee.' Her other hand plays with one skinny plait hanging over her shoulder.

'Is there anything to see in the town?' I ask.

'Yes. Here is the Presidential Palace, Nossa Senhora da Luz Church, and the Market Square.' She circles the sights with a red biro that is chewed at the end. 'And Cultural Centre here. Is close today.'

Back in London, when I looked at one of the unsent sun-bleached postcards of Cape Verde's beaches and palm trees, I reflected on the ten scattered islands, some as dry as the Sahara. Theodor Vogel, botanist on a British expedition to Africa in 1841, had said of the archipelago: '*One might believe that after the formation of the world, a quantity of useless surplus stones was cast into the sea.*'

Were they useless before the Portuguese arrived in 1462, when they were uninhabited? Too dry to support life? Was this the reason why more Cape Verdeans live abroad than on their home islands? Or have they never had sufficient income to support the population once slavery was abolished? I comfort myself with the thought that at least cruise-ship tourism boosts their meagre economy now.

The escudos I receive in change for the postcards look more exotic than the cards, carrying images of birds, old sailing ships and sea turtles, while the notes feature both a presidential-looking man and black slaves carrying rocks on their heads. Hadn't the wheel been invented by then? The note depicts a whole history in numismatics. At over one hundred escudos to a euro, the change is worthless to us: 'a quantity of useless surplus coins'.

The market is closed, except for a solitary stall run by an

engaging man selling leather belts and bags, locally beaded according to his handwritten sign hanging from the belt rack. He is persuading passengers of the appeal of his leatherware as mementos.

If there had been a port talk about the slave trade we would have learned all about Cape Verde's role and its Portuguese colonisation. Displayed on panels surrounding the marketplace are large blue ceramic tiles, azulejos, covered with hand-painted scenes depicting life in the colony during the nineteenth century. I am struck by one that shows two bare-foot black women in local dress, each carrying what appears to be a large sack of coal on her head, the pair linking arms to steady themselves like yoked oxen, followed a short distance behind by a top-hatted white man holding a whip. We would have been told about the women slaves carrying Welsh coal at a time when hundreds of thousands of tons were stored on Cape Verde to refuel the countless steamships that stopped during their Atlantic crossings in the 1800s. Due to the prevailing westerly winds blowing on to Cape Verde it was ideally placed in the Atlantic shipping lanes to re-supply ships, especially laden slave ships en route to North and South America.

It was the trade winds and the ocean currents that determined the direction of Atlantic slave trade voyages – clockwise wind and currents in the north, anti-clockwise in the south. Empty slave vessels started out from Europe and America in the north, loaded their slave cargo in Africa then sailed across with the southern winds to Brazil, North America and Europe. It formed a figure of eight.

I point out the blue tile to Tom.

'And this was at a time when women in England were considered too weak to hold down the job of secretary. Secretaries were all men.'

'Well, don't forget that they had to carry ledgers and quill pens and all that sort of thing, dear. Women would have fainted if they'd've been made to do that,' says Tom.

Mindel Hotel is a flaky, flat-fronted blue building in need of refurbishment. There is no lift, or maybe the lift isn't working; either way, we climb the stairs to the fourth floor. The large room at the top with its dark-wood bar, backed by bottles of spirits and imported beer, opens out onto an unshaded terrace with a view of the port. The sun hits the floor, radiating fiery heat in all directions. A ceiling fan rotates too slowly to produce a breeze. How glad I am to be wearing just three items of clothing. Behind the bar sits a filter coffee machine in which the treacly liquid is continuously heated. A young, slender bartender stands in unbecoming brown trousers and shirt with the hotel's blue logo on the breast pocket. He speaks little English. Still, he only needs to understand mime to dispense two coffees. It's good to get rid of our escudos, leaving what looks like a generous tip but which is probably worth tuppence. We are the only people in the bar; indeed, in the entire hotel as far as we can make out. The coffees are undrinkable. Hot, but as bitter as Mindelo's history. I manage to finish mine by adding tooth-aching quantities of sugar. Tom swallows his like medicine, making the face of an infant who's been made to swallow polio drops by having his nose squeezed. The young man looks pleased to be occupied, clearing away our cups and wiping the bar down several times. We echo his 'Tchaus', and take the stairs to the street.

Back on board, I first visit Mr Richardson to find out the results of his chest X-ray.

'It cost a heck of a lot,' says Vera. 'Three hundred and fifty euros just for the X-rays, and there was a lot of hanging about waiting. It'd've been quicker at our local hospital in Worcester.

Then there was the cost of the cab there and back. Anyway, we've got the X-rays. Now where... did I... put them?'

'In front of you, Vera. There. On the table,' says Mr Richardson, who is slumped in bed looking pale and unwell.

Mrs Richardson hands me the large brown envelope.

'Is there a letter from the doctor?'

'I don't know. No-one mentioned it. Should they have?'

'I was expecting one, but never mind. I'll check your X-rays properly down in the Medical Centre, then I'll ring you.'

It must have been twenty years since I'd regularly interpreted chest X-rays as a junior doctor in chest medicine. I could remember the principles but I could no longer consider myself competent in the detail. I'd ordered the X-rays but hadn't requested the radiologist's report. They might have guessed I would want it, but then, I hadn't asked. I stick the X-rays up on the light boxes. There is clouding in the right lung. I can't be sure whether it represents pneumonia or bronchitis, or something else.

I ring the hospital and ask to speak to the radiologist, slowly and loudly as though I am talking to a small child with poor hearing.

A man's voice comes on the line. 'Olá.'

'Do you speak English?'

'Inglês? Não.'

'SHIP'S DOCTOR. DOCTOR TAYLOR. SHIP *SEA RAINBOW*. MR RICHARDSON'S CHEST X-RAYS. REPORT PLEASE. REPORT TO SHIP.'

I am hoping some of the words are similar in Portuguese, but then it's an unusual language, sounding a bit like Russian to the untrained ear. Not quite a romance language. I reassure myself, however, that the report's medical terminology, based on Latin and Greek, is going to be similar in most European languages.

'Si. Si.'

I read out the fax number, but as I don't know Portuguese numbers, I can't be sure he's understood. I call the port agent, Joseph, and ask him to obtain the report.

'As quickly as possible, because we leave at six, and I want to tell Mr Richardson his result and organise treatment.' Or repatriation if the diagnosis is unmanageable on board.

Twenty minutes later Joseph rings back. 'The radiologist says could you fax him the request for the report.'

'But I've just *spoken* to him personally half an hour ago.'

'He says he must have it in writing.'

Of course he does. We would in the UK too.

The Medical Centre doesn't have a fax machine. I run the letter up to reception and asked the receptionist to ring me when they get a reply.

Then I ring Mr Richardson to explain the delay.

While I'm waiting, Liz and I do the gastro phoning. Numbers are reducing. I feel a bout of gripes starting. I can't have a third attack. I simply can't. I'll be a case. I hold my breath, gently massage my stomach, and hang on.

A crew member is waiting. Rosa, short, in her early forties, black hair tied back, sitting in her blue and white stewardess uniform, complains of an itchy rash that has started that morning. She shows me the tiny red bumps, mainly on her abdomen and back; lots of them. A few have started to appear on her face and some look as though they are forming tiny blisters. She has a fever. Chickenpox. I ask her if she's had it before. She doesn't know.

'If you ring your mother, ask her if *she* remembers you

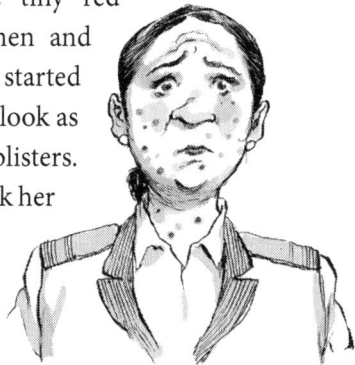

having had it as a child. Chickenpox. Varicella. I don't know the name in Filipino. I'll write it down for you.' If Rosa was having a recurrent episode, it might indicate a problem with her immune system, rarely HIV.

'You gonna gib me antibiotics?'

'No, Rosa. Antibiotics won't do anything. It's a virus. Your body will kill the virus. An antibiotic won't.'

'What you gonna gib me?' She already looks disappointed.

'Well, everything for your symptoms. Paracetamol for fever, calamine lotion and antihistamines for the rash. You can put the calamine lotion on your spots as many times as you want to and the antihistamine tablet you take three times a day. They might make you feel drowsy, but at least you'll be able to sleep at night. OK?'

Rosa hesitates. 'But can I go to work now?'

'*No.* You're infectious for seven days. Other people can catch it from you. I'll sign you off work for a week. You'll need to let your manager know… Liz, hand me some sick notes please.'

'What's Rosa got?' she asks as she stands by the door.

'Chickenpox.'

'Ah, I thought it might be. A lot of Filipino crew get it. They don't seem to have it as children. Don't know why. I'll bleep Oleg to sort out an empty cabin…' Liz comes into the consulting room. 'Listen. You can't go back to your cabin, Rosa. I'll tell you which cabin to go to. Meals from room service, and you'll have to ask friends to leave any of your things outside the door for you. Do you understand? You – can't – go – back – to – your – own – cabin,' Liz repeats.

'Oh. Which cabin I'm habing?'

'I'll tell you in a minute or two. Stay here until you've got your new cabin number and medication.' Liz steps back into the nurses' office.

'I'll come and see you every day,' I say. 'I've had chickenpox myself, so I won't catch it from you. Normally you can only have it once; after that you're immune.' I guess the word 'immune' will be similar in Filipino. I don't tell her that one of my patients has had it three times.

I remember my partner in General Practice telling me that a patient of hers – a young adult – had died in hospital of varicella pneumonia. It must have been in the 1970s. Although there is less than a one in ten thousand chance of this, any doctor who sees a patient die of something treatable, or avoidable, will always remember it and be wary. If the doctor was responsible for the patient, they will never forget, may never forgive themselves. I wasn't going to let even this rare complication happen to Rosa.

Rosa is not happy. 'Can my friends bisit?'

'Sorry, no – because you can pass the infection to them if they haven't had chickenpox themselves. No visitors, except nurse or doctor. But you should be out in seven days. Ask your friends to get you some books or magazines to read and there will be a TV in the cabin. You can rest.'

'I can hab a shower?'

'Yes, you can shower whenever you want to, but not too hot. You'll be more itchy if you're hot.'

Rosa's eyes and face redden. She looks as if she is going to cry.

'Don't worry. You'll be alright.' I put my hand on hers.

'I don't like be sick.' Is she worried about her sickness record for the next contract?

'Listen. You're in four-one-two. It'll be unlocked,' Liz calls out. Rosa leaves with medication and instructions. 'She must have caught it off *someone*. But we haven't seen anyone with chickenpox. Maybe we should get her cabin mates in for a check-up – though they'd obviously notice if they'd had it.'

'Not necessarily. Some people only get a few spots and don't feel ill, so they think they're insect bites and ignore them.' I comb both hands through my hair. The incubation period is about a fortnight and as this is day ten of the cruise, someone could have passed it on then disembarked in the UK.

'Oh hell. We don't want a chickenpox outbreak on top of noro. That would be the living end. I'd better notify Rosa's cabin companions and get their cabin fumigated.'

'Right, let's call them in while you're about it. At least we can tell them what to look out for and what to report. Where's Coralie?' I ask.

'Ashore. She should be back anytime. By the way, you better tell the Captain about Rosa, and Dr Wallis.'

Mr Richardson's X-ray report is back.

The report states 'uma área de consolidação no lobo inferior direito'. My eye falls on the word 'consolidação'. Right lower lobe consolidation. Pneumonia.

I collect the thermometer, sphygmomanometer (blood pressure machine), stethoscope and blood oxygen saturation device. As I climb the stairs, I hear the ship's engines groaning and feel the ship start to move, like riding on the back of a huge elephant. We are leaving Mindelo.

'There is a patch of pneumonia in the right lung,' I explain to Mr Richardson and Vera; a patch sounding not nearly as bad as a whole lobe. 'It's on the report from the hospital, but don't worry, I'm sure we can get you right.'

Kneeling next to his bunk I examine him. His temperature and pulse are still too high, oxygen saturation and blood pressure lower than is healthy. In General Practice I had learned the hard way to treat the ill elderly like sick babies – with extra care and attention, because their resilience and resistance to infection are not as sturdy as in younger adults and their condition could deteriorate rapidly.

I move the chair next to his bed. 'Your temperature is still high and the oxygen in your blood is rather low. I want to take you down to our hospital to start antibiotics intravenously and give you some oxygen. That way everything will work faster and get on top of the infection sooner. Would that be OK?'

'Does he have to go down to the hospital? Couldn't he have it done here – in the cabin?' Vera asks.

'I'd rather keep a close eye on him, make sure the antibiotics suit him, and make sure he's improving.'

'What do you think, John?' Vera asks.

'Whatever the doctor says…' John's voice is faint and croaky.

I ring Liz and explain the plan.

'Bring his overnight things as well as his medication,' I tell Vera.

Coralie is in the Medical Centre attending to Mr Wayfield's inhalation. I can hear her chatting to him. 'Is that orright? Not too tight? Just sit there and breathe easy. I'm nearby if you want me. I'll be back in a mo.'

She comes into the office. Liz tells her about Mr Richardson. 'Can you do the gastros while I fetch him?' Liz grabs the wheelchair.

Coralie looks haggard. Can I smell alcohol again? She goes back in to check Mr Wayfield, then takes the gastro notes into a side ward.

The puttering of the nebuliser stops.

'How're you doing now?' I say, standing in front of Mr Wayfield.

'Better. It couldn't have been pneumonia, could it?'

Surely he hasn't overheard our conversation.

'No,' I say. 'I checked your chest for pneumonia several times. You hadn't got a fever, and antibiotics made no difference. Your cough has been persistent because you have a tendency to asthma, so your breathing tubes have overreacted. The inhalations are calming them down.'

I'm not sure whether my explanation would pass a viva in

chest medicine. Returning to my consulting room, I make sure the door is shut.

'Captain Strom, we have a case of chickenpox. One of the stewardesses. She's confined in four-one-two.'

'Chickenpox? You're quite *sure*?'

'Yes. It's absolutely textbook.'

'Brazilian Port Health are not going to like this. No-one else has it?' He sounds irritated.

'No. Not at present. We're checking her cabin companions as soon as we get hold of them.'

'I see. E-mail the Heads of Departments and ask them to warn all crew to report any spots to the Medical Centre.'

Oh no. The Medical Centre will be full of crew with mosquito bites, warts and acne.

Liz wheels Mr Richardson into the hospital ward. He is wearing an oxygen mask. Liz inserts the intravenous line. Coralie has started a set of observation records and puts his clothes into the bedside locker. I check the dose and frequency of the IV antibiotics and inject the first dose, followed by IV paracetamol. We agree on the instructions for ensuing doses and IV fluids. Coralie records it all in his notes and I leave them to it.

Back in the office with them I propose a plan. 'I want Mr Richardson to stay in the hospital tonight for observation and for IV "antibees". We can have a rota – split the night into three and I'll do a third.'

'No-o. We're not doing that,' Coralie says. 'I tell you, we haven't got the staff to look after anyone in hospital all night. Not just for antibiotics. He can have them up in his cabin.'

'Coralie, I don't want a seventy-eight-year-old man with a high fever, low sats and pneumonia somewhere where we can't easily see him or do regular obs. He needs to be watched at least overnight to see how he goes. If I'd been sure he had pneumonia before we left Mindelo, I'd have repatriated him. He's not safe in the cabin.'

'So, how often do you want his obs done?' asks Liz, not looking at Coralie.

'At least hourly.'

'We can't keep up hourly obs all ruddy night. We won't get any sleep, and we've got another day tomorrow.' Coralie drums her hands on the desk to the beat of her protest.

'OK. But he *needs* watching overnight. Who's on in the morning?' I ask.

'I am,' says Coralie.

I propose a rota for the three of us, with me working the first shift from eleven p.m. to two a.m. Liz and Coralie do not look enthusiastic. I'd rather stay up until two, then get my head down for the rest of the night. There's only one of me. I leave Liz and Coralie to sort out their shifts, no doubt grumbling about the harsh regime.

In the Age of Sail the only treatment the ship's doctor could offer a feverish patient was immersion in a bath of cold sea water or blood-letting, either of which could easily worsen the patient's condition or even cause their death.

I am grateful that even in the middle of a vast ocean we have modern medicine at our fingertips and science to back us up.

~⚓~

'Mindelo? There's nothing there. *And* everything was shut. A complete waste of time. I came back after half an hour. More things to do on board. Fancy stopping on a Sunday! Daft. Waste of our time,' Reginald repeats himself over his steak, grunting.

'Well, we liked the toon. Nice and quiet, so it was. We were away at the tropical gardens to the back there. The wee coloured birds were lovely. I don't know what they were – black with yellow chests,' says Mary, waving her hands down her front. 'They aren't in our bird book. We were hoping to see the Cape

Verde Warbler. Only so big,' Mary opened her thumb and index finger, 'but such a beautiful song. They're endangered, so they are.'

'The black and yellow ones stayed up in the palm trees, eating dates,' Jim added. 'I'd have liked to know what they were.'

'I'll search online,' Derek says.

'We didn't feel very safe in town,' says Pam, 'did we, Derek, even though we were on the tour. Our guide told everyone to keep belongings out of sight and to take off our jewellery.' Pam moves her watch up her arm.

'But then everyone is so poor. No wonder they'll pinch something if they get half a chance,' Derek says.

'It's the same in London,' Tom quips.

'A lot of them are descended from slaves. Apparently, it was a big slave transit place. They worked the sugar cane, although we couldn't see anywhere to grow it. Too dry and dusty,' says Derek.

'It's maybe on another island,' says Jim.

'Really nice tour. We saw the President's House, the church, and the market. Only it wasn't open,' Pam continues.

'Did you see the blue ceramic tiles?' I ask.

'They were really beautiful. All that history and artistry,' says Pam, beaming.

I do not disabuse her of the beauty of the slave women driven like donkeys. I don't want to sound like Mother Theresa.

'Inland is just a desert... a few small farms. So *dry – parched*. What they grow I've no idea. We did see some goats, didn't we, Derek?'

'Goats and dogs,' says Derek. 'The guide said Sahara's sand has been blowing over the island for centuries, millennia. We saw massive sand dunes, didn't we? Higher than a house,' says Derek, raising his hand.

'But then it's only six hundred miles from the African coast,' says Tom, 'so clearly the weather would be like Africa.'

'They laid on a smashing lunch. Near a big beach. What was it called, Derek – that beach?'

'Fish Bay, or something like that.'

'And there was a Spanish band.'

'Portuguese,' says Derek.

'That's what I mean. Terrific music – a singer, guitarist, and another one… drums. Lots of fish and meat, rice, salad and a sort of custard tart with fruit. You could just help yourself.' Pam licks the corners of her mouth.

'I hear there's a passenger with double pneumonia,' Mary was addressing me.

'Just single pneumonia,' I say, wondering if I'd already disclosed too much.

'Och, dearie me. How is he?' How did she know it was a 'he'? Careful.

'Not too bad,' I say.

'Poor soul. Will he be alright?' Mary leans towards me.

'I certainly hope so,' I say, as though it is nothing to do with me. The more detail I give the more the story will be inflated as it flies around the ship, until it turns into an epidemic of pneumonic plague caused by the ship's air-conditioning system and so untreatable that death inevitably follows, filling the morgue and all the spare cabins with corpses that are being kept secret.

─────⚓─────

When Tom and I arrive at the Pool Bar the dancefloor is full. Lee is singing Roy Orbison's *Pretty Woman*, not quite with the distinctive, rich sound of the 'Big O', but near enough. I've had a weak spot for Roy Orbison since I saw him in concert in Melbourne in the 1960s. He'd followed a group called The Flies, or was it The Insects? The teenage girls screamed all the way through the group's performance, but when Orbison came on stage the hall fell completely silent. He could sing.

Worming our way into the crowd, we find a spot where we can do our 'wiggle'. A jive is not only impossible in that crush, but contrary to health and safety. Besides I don't want to appear to be drumming up business.

It's Lee's last number so he hands over to the Confections with a small fanfare and a generous smile. The duo and Lee appear to be on excellent terms. Liz is seated at her customary table in her tropical uniform, waiting for Lee to join her. A few minutes later they leave together.

As I update Tom on the day's news and my night-shift duty for Mr Richardson, he watches a premier league football match featuring Arsenal on the TV in the corner of the bar. When he responds to my report it's with 'oh' and 'mm'.

Dave sings an Elvis number from 1960: *Are You Lonesome Tonight?* The dance hosts rise at the sound of a waltz. Edward chooses Eleanor, Brian takes Lesley, and Peter comes over to me.

'Would you care for this dance?' Always the gentleman.

'Is it OK if I do this one?' I ask Tom, remembering our previous testy exchange.

'Yes, sure.' He is preoccupied with the football, and besides, I suspect he can't face another whisk and weave.

Peter holds out his hand to guide me onto the floor. He is a natural dancer, light on his feet, precise, and with a gentle but firm lead that means my feet move where Peter intends them to go, without any feeling that I am being driven. However, he is strictly a ballroom dancer, lacking the disinhibition Tom displays for an outlandish jive or an eccentric hip-swinging 'wiggle'.

We chat about our day as we sway effortlessly across the floor, performing a perfect reverse turn at each end.

'I escorted one of the tours,' says Peter. 'You ought to put your name down. You don't have to pay for the tour. You just need to register at the Tours Desk.'

'Yes, one of the nurses told me about it, but I haven't done it yet. Which tour?' He has speckled grey eyes – kind, with a touch of sadness in them. I can feel his wiry, athletic shoulder through his jacket.

'Panoramic Cape Verde. We walked around Mindelo, then went miles across the island. There was a lunch stop too, with music – very pleasant.'

'Our table companions were on that one.'

'Who are they?'

'Pam and Derek. Rather a big couple.'

'Mm, I think I know who you mean. They've got good appetites, haven't they? How's your man with pneumonia?' Peter asks in the middle of a chassé.

I wince inwardly. This Chinese whisper has travelled faster than a Japanese bullet train. Did it originate with Mr Wayfield? Has confidentiality been lax in the Medical Centre?

'Not too bad. Should be OK.' I look over my left shoulder, as we complete a seamless whisk and weave. I feel transported. To dance is a joy. The music stops. Peter guides me back to my seat on his hand.

The next number is *D-I-V-O-R-C-E*, made famous by Tammy Wynette. Lesley, Eleanor and Pat are on the floor doing a line dance. Edward and Brian join them. Gradually some more women and a couple of men get up. Tom remains engrossed in the football match, so I join the group. Following their routine doesn't look difficult as the same sequence of ten steps is repeated over and again, but that doesn't stop me getting the moves mixed up. Give me a proper ballroom dance any day. Still, any kind of dance is preferable to watching football.

Dave is on to *Darling Save The Last Dance for Me*, a 1960 Drifters' number. The beat is perfect for cha-cha.

'Come on Tom, *let's* do this one. It's a salsa,' I say, knowing Tom feels foolish trying those fast little cha-cha steps. A salsa we can do to the same beat.

'No,' he says, eyes glued to the TV, 'I'll do the next one.'

I've heard that before.

Honesty by Billy Joel follows. Ironic.

'Come on then.' I touch his hand. 'It's a Why Dance.'

'Do you *want* to do this one?' Tom glances at me, then back to the TV.

'*Yes.* Oh, come *on.*'

Tom takes off his jacket. He never dances in his jacket. It cramps his style. But as there are two TVs in the bar, one on each side of the room, he can follow the game whichever way we're facing. Although we are in close hold, it doesn't feel like an intimate dance, more like a watching-the-football-from-the-floor dance.

'I'm going down to the hospital to see that patient.'

'You've got a patient at this time of night? Did your bleep go?' Tom looks at his watch. 'It's nearly eleven!'

'No, I *told* you – we've got a passenger in the hospital overnight. He's the one with pneumonia. I told you. I'm down in the hospital now till two o'clock, then one of the nurses will take over from me.'

'Do you mean you're staying up till two in the morning?'

'*I said* – we agreed that the three of us would split the night shift and I'd do eleven to two, three hours. Anyway, I have to go.' As I leave, Tom's eyes flick back to the match.

Liz is sitting in a chair at the foot of Mr Richardson's bed. He is either sleeping or unconscious.

'How is he?' I whisper.

'Everything's stable,' she says.

I pick up his observation chart. His oxygen level and blood pressure are still lower than I would like, but it is night-time, when the levels drop naturally. His breathing is quicker than normal under his oxygen mask, but not laboured.

'Has he been awake?'

'Yes. He woke up for a drink about half an hour ago.'

'Antibiotic?'

'Yep – on the chart – under ten p.m. See?' Liz stands and taps her pen on the entry.

'Where's the next dose?'

'No. It's alright. You go to bed. I'll stay.'

'*No.* I said I'd split the night with you two.' I stand, feet planted.

'No, honestly. It's easier for us. We can catch up. There's only one of you.'

I am longing to go to bed. I don't argue.

Mr Richardson mutters something unintelligible in his sleep. We glance across at him.

'Coralie's fine about it. I'm doing till three, then Coralie'll take over till eight, then I'll come back on and she can go to bed.'

I can't imagine Coralie being 'fine' about anything to do with this arrangement.

I leave with a warm appreciation of our small team.

When I get into the cabin Tom isn't there. I lay my uniform on the armchair in donning order as if I am a firefighter ready to jump into it and shin down a slippery pole in an instant.

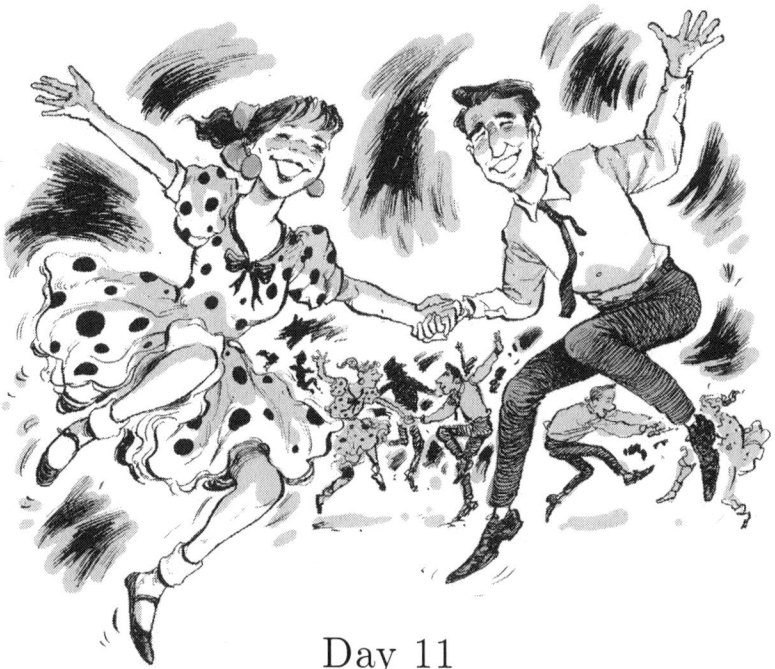

Day 11

Mandy

'Thanks for doing my shift last night. How's our patient?' I ask Coralie.

'Fine.' She is holding the phone in one hand, looking at the gastro notes with the other.

'Wasn't Liz doing this morning?'

'She'll be down in a mo.' For the first time since the disciplinary Coralie looks me briefly in the eye, then continues ringing the gastros.

Mr Richardson is sitting up looking alert with a tray of unfinished tea and toast on his bedtable, crumbs down his pyjama top. Vera sits beside him.

'I think I'm a bit better,' Mr Richardson says. 'Do I have to keep these things up my nose?'

I look at the monitor. His oxygen level has risen nicely. His observation chart shows that his blood pressure is also near normal.

'No, I think we can dispense with those now. Your oxygen reading is better. Let me take those tubes out, and we'll see how you go without them. All being well, we might be able to discharge you today.'

'That'd be good. This bed's blooming uncomfortable.' It is a good sign when a sick patient starts complaining.

'You can sit out in the armchair this morning. I'll get nurse to help.' I turn to Vera. 'He's doing well.'

'He looks better. A healthier colour. Did you say he can come out today?'

'Hopefully. We'll just see what he's like without oxygen, and whether he's steady on his feet. We'll know in about an hour or so.'

'In that case I'll go up on deck for some air and come down later, shall I, John?' Vera says.

Liz arrives and takes over while I start surgery.

Rosa's three cabin companions are waiting to be checked. None of them know if they've had chickenpox. I press them all to ask their mothers if they are in phone contact, and to put anything Rosa wants outside her cabin door. They are under strict instructions to report back if they develop a rash or fever.

I return to Mr Richardson.

'It's alright for him to go to the bathroom, isn't it?' Liz checks.

'See what he's like on his feet first… You can take your intravenous set with you,' I tell Mr Richardson. 'I'm sure I've seen an IV stand on wheels somewhere around here. You know, to hang the IV fluids on.'

Fifteen minutes later Liz comes out to the office.

'How was he?' I ask.

'Good. He's pretty steady on his legs.'

'Sats?'

'Ninety-seven percent.'

'That'll do fine. Let's get him discharged. I want him to have another twenty-four hours of IV antibees, then he can go on oral if he's making progress. Take the drip down and leave the IV line in. Call me when he's ready.'

'I don't like here. I can't see my friends and no window,' Rosa pouts. She has been allocated an inside passenger cabin. That's mean. She is covered in spots and looks miserable. Her hair sticks up where she's been lying on it. Her temperature is high but her chest is clear.

'Are you taking paracetamol?'

'Yes.'

'When was the last time?'

'Yesterday.'

'It only lasts four hours, so you need to take it regularly if you're hot. It will help you feel better. Are you very itchy?'

'Not bery much. Do I hab to stop here seben days?'

'Yes. Because you're infectious for seven days. But now you've only got six days,' I say, trying to be cheerful.

'It's so long time. Can't I hab a window?' Her eyes well up with tears.

I touch her arm. 'Let's see. I'll ask Oleg.'

At the daily gastro meeting I report no new cases and six passengers discharged. The total passengers and crew confined is now under zero point two percent.

'So, can we step back to Code Orange? What do you say, Doctor?' Captain Strom asks.

The responsibility.

'Well, it's looking positive. The number of new cases has reduced significantly, and we're now discharging every day.'

'Right – step down to Code Orange. Heads of Departments, let all your staff know.'

Goodness. That's precipitous. I'd prefer a lot more dilly-dallying.

There is a palpable sigh of relief from the Maître d', who's been struggling to find enough waiters to serve the buffet food, the dining tables and cabin service for the gastros. His staff have been working harder and having even less time off than usual. They start at six a.m. and finish at midnight. Those on duty for room service are up all night. Some staff from other departments, such as entertainment, have been recruited to help serve afternoon teas in order to give the waiters a break. It means that the crew member in khaki shirt and shorts, who organises the dolphin race and deck quoits, also serves the scones, jam and clotted cream.

I bleep Oleg, the Hotel Manager, to ask him for an outside cabin for Rosa.

'Sorry. I haven't got a free outside cabin. The ship's full.'

'Really? Well, if one becomes free will you let me know?'

'Sure.'

I ring Rosa. 'Oleg doesn't have an outside cabin, but as soon as there's one free, he'll let me know.'

'Oh, OK.' At least she doesn't burst into tears.

***

In the hospital Mr Richardson is in a red dressing gown, ready to return to his cabin.

'Take it easy today, but don't stay in bed. Move about the cabin. Only go on deck if it's warm, and then just for, say, half an hour. We'll be coming up to give you your antibiotics every eight hours anyway. Do you think you could come down to see *me* tomorrow morning?'

'Yes, I should think so.' He looks at Vera for confirmation.

'If not just let us know and I'll come to you. Can you take him up in the wheelchair, Liz?'

'No. I'm alright to go on my own. Honestly,' Mr Richardson says.

'Not in pyjamas and dressing gown. You'll frighten the passengers. Come down independently tomorrow.'

***

It is midday. The loudspeakers hiss: 'This is Captain Strom with the noon report from the navigational bridge. Our present position is fourteen point four degrees north by thirty-one point two degrees west. The wind is a light north-easterly with a gentle breeze of five knots. Our present speed is twelve knots, and we have been steaming two hundred and seventy-six nautical miles from Sao Vicente in the Cape Verde Islands, which is three hundred and seventeen statute miles. This leaves one thousand one hundred and four nautical miles to go to Fortaleza, Brazil, equivalent to one thousand two hundred and seventy statute miles. The air temperature is twenty-seven degrees centigrade, which is eighty degrees Fahrenheit. The sea temperature is twenty-five degrees centigrade, seventy-seven degrees Fahrenheit. The barometric pressure is one hundred and two point eight millibars, so we can expect a sunny day today on our way to Fortaleza in Brazil. Due to a temporary shortage of fresh water, we ask that all passengers and crew conserve water as much as possible. Avoid drinking the water from your cabin taps. The situation will ease at the next port of call. I will keep you informed. Have a very pleasant afternoon, ladies and gentlemen.'

One hundred and fifty years previously, in the Age of Sail, there was no means of keeping drinking water fresh on long journeys. The water became slimy and turned the sailors' stomachs. Consequently, a crewman's rations included one gallon of beer daily and half a pint of rum. However, as the beer turned sour, rum became the only unspoiled drink available. No wonder sailors fell into the sea. On today's ships drinking water is freshly desalinated and refrigerated.

'This epidemic won't leave us alone,' Liz says as I walk into the Medical Centre. 'There's one new case and one observation.'

'No... *again*? Are either of them for me?'

'The observation case could be seen. He's a bit complicated. Mr Sheehan – Ron Sheehan, five-six-seven. He's a regular. Comes on board for months at a time.'

'Right. I'll see him now before we start. I've just about got time. By the way, did you hear the noon report?'

'The water rationing?' Liz looks at me, one eyebrow raised.

'Yes. Why do we have to conserve suddenly?'

'Apparently the water we took on in Mindelo was contaminated. I don't know whether with oil or bugs or what, but it's not usable.'

'How do you know?'

'I overheard Sergei talking about it at breakfast. It'll just mean using bottled water at the tables and I suppose the desalination plant will have to work overtime to provide more drinking water.'

'I thought we already used bottled water at the tables.'

'No. It's only iced tap water. The tap water's meant to be perfectly drinkable, but it's not now.' Liz turns back to the filing cabinet.

Mr Sheehan has had an episode of abdominal pain, nausea and one bout of diarrhoea on the previous day. He feels unwell, is off his food and still nauseated. His temperature is 37.4°C, which is tricky. It's not high enough to be called a fever, but as 37°C is deemed the upper limit of normal, it isn't entirely normal either. Who knows whether it is on its way up or down.

'Hello, Doc. You're new. How're you finding it?' Mr Sheehan, a seasoned cruiser, says. 'I thought I'd eaten something that disagreed with me, though I've got a pretty strong stomach, I can tell you. I never suffer with me stomach. But I went on one of them tours yesterday and had the buffet lunch. I thought the fish tasted a bit... old – not *off*, but not that fresh, but then my mate ate the same thing and *he's* alright. Anyhow, you know, I thought I'd better report it. I've seen how bugs can whip round a ship.'

As he speaks, I see that his face is lop-sided and his speech slightly slurred, as though he's had a stroke.

'I hear you're a frequent cruiser,' I say, sinking into the armchair next to his bunk.

'You could say that. From April to September, I do back-to-back cruises for the whole summer, then for the rest of the year I'm at home, in Godmanchester, near Huntingdon.'

'Can I ask you – your face looks slightly uneven on one side, and I notice your speech is affected. Are they new things?'

'No, no, no. I was in a car crash eight years ago. A bad crash. I was unconscious for three weeks. Had twelve months of rehab to get walking again... My wife – um – was in the car.' He pauses. 'She didn't make it.' He pauses again. His eyes redden and his bottom lip puckers. His breath quickens.

'I'm sorry,' I murmur, touching his arm. He squeezes his lips tightly together.

'No. It's alright.' He moves his arm away, takes a deep breath and continues. 'I knew that I'd got a second chance, so I sold our house and bought a houseboat. I've got a cracking view across the marina. And there's all the water birds – I love all that. I spend the rest of the money on cruising. It's not a bad life, you know. It'll do until I go out boots first.' He holds my gaze.

'Well, it's good that you called us, but it doesn't quite sound like gastroenteritis. Have you had norovirus before?'

'Have I *had* it? I'll say *I have*. What a business *that* was. It was coming out at both ends. I thought I was exploding. No, this is nothing like that. I don't want it either, I can tell you.'

'If you've had it before it does give you *some* immunity. At least if you do get it again it shouldn't be as bad as the first time. But we'll just have to see. Stay put and either nurse or I will ring you tomorrow morning for a report. I'll leave you some anti-sickness pills you can take if you're nauseated and you can order light food from room service if you have an appetite. Don't force yourself though.'

'OK. Thanks, Doc. Where are you from then?'

'From London – my practice is in the East End.'

'I know the East End. My parents lived in Hackney for about ten years. Dad worked as a printer in Fleet Street. And I'm an Arsenal fan.'

'How awful. My husband's an Arsenal fundamentalist. For goodness' sake don't tell him you support Arsenal. You two'll never be off the subject.' I peer at my watch under the edge of the plastic glove. 'Saying that, I've got to get on or I'll be in trouble.'

Predictably, I am late back to the Medical Centre. Liz has departed to do the water testing, then she'll be off duty, leaving Coralie in charge. From the consulting room I can hear her slapping things down in the office as usual, muttering to herself, and being short with patients.

Mrs Wilson enters with Mr Wilson a few steps behind. I am surprised that he's agreed to come with her. 'Good to see you both,' I say as I fetch another chair.

I check Mrs Wilson's blood pressure. 'One hundred and fifty-six over ninety-eight. That *is* improving – no doubt about it. Now, what about you two?'

'Well, you said to bring Neil in.'

'So, how are things?'

'He's still drinking too much,' Mrs Wilson pronounces the guilty verdict.

'But I've cut right down,' is Mr Wilson's defence.

'From what? From one bottle of whisky a day to half? You ask the doctor how much you should be drinking.'

'How much *are* you drinking, Mr Wilson?'

'She always exaggerates. I have a few tots.'

'Poof – *a few tots*,' exclaims Ruby. 'Tell her the truth.'

'Is the drinking a problem?' I venture.

'I'll say it is,' Ruby says. 'Tell her about that time when you were cruel to the dog. It was unforgiveable.' I do not want to hear about Mr Wilson's animal cruelty.

'Only Ruby thinks it's a problem. I've got friends who drink a lot more than me.'

'Friends? Those boring old drunks down The Tavern? He drinks every night, Doctor. I've put up with it for years, but he's getting worse.'

'Mr Wilson, it obviously *is* an issue, at least for Mrs Wilson. Do you think you can cut down? Have three or four non-drinking days a week, say? Start drinking later in the evening? Have smaller measures? Miss rounds?'

'I don't know.' He looks at his hands. Acute Deficiency of Motivation is my diagnosis.

'There'll be a local alcohol service that can help you when you get home. I can write a letter to your GP, if you like.'

'Would you? That would be really helpful, Doctor,' says Ruby, with a look of exasperation in Mr Wilson's direction.

'Another thing, Doctor.'

'Yes, Mr Wilson.'

'Do you stock Viagra?'

Ruby's head shakes barely perceptibly.

'Sorry, no, we don't.'

Lorenz, one of the bar crew, is back with his urticaria.

'How's this nettle rash?' I ask, examining his face and arms.

'A bit better, but it's still there. See?' He shows me his upper arm, bearing large wheals. 'When I get it wet it's worse, so *itchy*. I try not to scratch, but I can't help it. I do it in my sleep.' He watches me running my fingers over the scratched areas to assess the rash, raised or flat, hard or soft. People who have rashes don't get touched, but I'm not going to catch anything and it is good practice to feel the skin of someone who may see themselves as untouchable.

'Have you had any patch testing?' I hold his arm in both hands.

'I don't know. What is it?' He watches my hands moving over his skin.

'It's a test for allergies. If you see a skin specialist, they can test small areas of your skin with different things to see if you're allergic to something.' I let go.

'No. I haven't done it. Not a specialist.'

'What about at home in the Philippines?'

'I don't have rashes when I'm at home.'

'So-o... you must be allergic to something on board.'

'I told the last doctor, but he only gave me cream,' Lorenz says, scratching his arm.

I rub my arm reflexively. I can read the last doctor's notes, but there are always things unwritten. Up to forty percent of a consultation doesn't end up in the patient's record.

'Let's get you patch-tested. They usually put the patches on one day, then read the results twenty-four or forty-eight hours later.' I felt confident that this procedure would be standard practice anywhere in the world. 'When does your contract finish?'

'Six munts.'

'Right. I'll organise for you to see a dermatologist in Rio. We're in port for three days, so there'll be time to do the test and get the results from the same clinic. I'll change your medication now to see if it'll be more helpful. Do you need extra cream?'

'I don't have nothing now.' Lorenz looks fed up.

'Don't run out. If you need more of anything, just come down and ask nurse. And no hot showers. Keep the water cool and the shower short.'

Coralie wordlessly gathers the medication from the pharmacy and hands it to Lorenz. She shuts the heavy grey metal door with a loud clack.

'Did anyone do the quiz today?' Derek asks, looking at Jim.

'We had a go, so we did,' Jim says.

'Question four was a teaser... um, *underwater* mountain in Europe? *Underwater?* I thought that was unfair. We decided it was in the Azores,' Derek says, his mouth full of liver pâté.

'Yes. They're all volcanic and mountainous... but which one?' Pam stares at the ceiling, sucking in her lip.

'It's Madeira,' Tom blurts out.

Everyone looks up.

Tom holds forth on the ninety-six percent of Madeira below the waterline, sounding as though he is giving a speech about policy at a trade union conference.

'Well, I never,' says Derek.

'Did anyone go to the fireman's lecture?' Jim says. 'I dinae ken after the Great Fire of London, insurance companies started their own fire brigades. Ye'd get a wee badge to fix onto your building, then if ye had a fire, ye tell the company and the brigade turns up and puts it out. If it's the wrong company, they'd away and leave your hame in flames. Can't have been funny,' Jim says, animated.

Mary asks me about her split fingernails when Reginald turns to Tom. 'I saw you drawing on deck. Were you a draughtsman?'

'The drawings are just, umm, studies for larger pieces of work. Ones I've planned for when I get home.' Tom looks down and resumes chewing each of his prawns the regulation fifty times.

Reginald nods, I suspect, without understanding.

'What sort of drawings do you do?' Pam asks.

'Well – er, the current series involves linear grids that are printed on glass, if that makes sense.'

I can see Pam's eyes glaze.

'He's an abstract artist,' I explain, as though Tom has an intellectual impairment.

Tom doesn't like to talk about his art. Most people don't understand or appreciate abstraction. Too much work for the viewer.

'Och, did ye no see the flying fish today?' Mary says.

'No. Where *were* they? *When?*' I feel cheated.

'All along the side, just gone eleven. Hundreds of them, and flying so far, I thought they'd never land. Like silver birds.'

'Did you see them, Tom, when you were on deck?' I ask. So lucky being on deck while I was in the bowels.

'No, I watched the match down in the cabin. Did anyone see the result?' He clearly meant Arsenal had won.

'Don't encourage him,' I say. How could he have missed the sun and flying fish for a football match?

'It's rock 'n' roll tonight. Right up your street. I hear you're great jivers,' Derek says.

'We do *real* jive – working-class jive. I've done it since I was fifteen in the church youth club. I used to dance with a girl called June Allan. She was four foot ten and the only one I could throw around,' Tom says. 'I suppose we *could* go if you want to, Ruth. We haven't been to any of the shows.'

'You *must* go. The ship's troupe are fabulous. The choreography is terrific, isn't it, Derek? Gorgeous costumes. We go to all the shows.'

'Do you know about the water problem?' Derek says, picking up and waggling one of the plastic water bottles on the table. 'What's this about?'

'I'm not sure. I'll see if I can catch the Chief Engineer.' I decide to avoid giving Liz's explanation to the table. The rumour would fly around the ship that the water had been poisoned and we'd all have to be air-lifted to Senegal for safety, then repatriated.

The cabaret lounge is packed. We thread our way along a row of seats to a partial view behind a pillar. It isn't good form for a Senior Officer to take a seat with a clear view of the stage that could be used by a passenger.

Starting with *Rock Around the Clock*, by Bill Haley and The Comets, the ship's company throw themselves into a dizzyingly fast jive. The women twirl their polka-dot skirts, jumping in bobby socks and white flatties, while the men spin them around and flip them over their heads, wearing tight black trousers, pencil ties and Brilliantined hair swooped up into a stiff quiff at the front. It is an adrenaline-charged performance. I am itching to join in, except that we – the 'great jivers' – wouldn't last thirty seconds. What am I talking about? Five seconds.

The audience tap their feet, clap their hands in rhythm and applaud loudly after each number. I am mesmerised. I have visions of myself being a professional dancer instead of a doctor. I'd be so famous. Lauded. Rich. Glamorous.

The dancers are flying to *Shake, Rattle 'n Roll* by Big Joe Turner, and bouncing all over the stage to *C'mon Everybody* by Eddie Cochran. Their feet are a blur to *Tutti Frutti* by Little Richard. So fast, Tom and I have branded it a St Vitus dance, and avoid doing it in case it brings on a conniption.

St Vitus had unusual responsibilities. He was the patron saint of dance *and* epilepsy. Why any saint troubled himself with dance when disabling untreatable epilepsy would have demanded so much more of his attention in the year 303 is hard to fathom.

The ship's dance troupe do the Lindy Hop: the men throw the women from behind over their shoulders, then roll over the bent backs of the women stooping in front of them. The whole group leap in the air, descending onto the stage in the splits with high-pitched yelps. They run off to tumultuous applause, whistles and bravos.

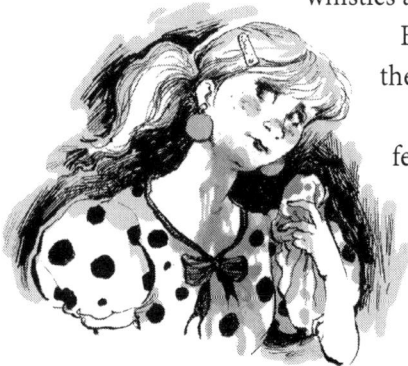

BEEP goes my bleeper. One of the dancers is injured.

Mandy, with her even features, blonde ponytail fastened in a spangled clip, holds a wadge of bloody material clamped to her chin. The front of her costume is layered in drying blood. A dance companion, also in her polka-dot skirt, is holding her hand.

'How did this happen?' I ask. As Coralie slowly peels off the blood-soaked dressing, I can see a two-centimetre long, deep cut on the point of Mandy's chin. She looks tearful. 'When I landed in the splits my head fell forward and I hit my chin on the stage. I didn't realise I'd done it until I saw blood all down my skirt... It won't scar, will it?' She is dependent on her good looks for her career.

'Mm, there will be a small scar, but actually,' I peer more closely at the wound, 'the cut is slightly back from the point of the chin so it won't really be noticed,' I hope. There is a brown mole just to the left of it and a sprinkling of freckles on her cheeks, so her face isn't flawless. Most people's faces aren't.

'Are you sure?'

'Well, I'll sew it as neatly as I can. I'll do invisible mending,' I say.

Mandy glances at her friend and they both look relieved.

The ship is rolling slightly, something I haven't noticed as I've become more accustomed to the movement. However, I am soon made acutely aware of it when I try to stitch Mandy's chin. The needle pierces the skin, the ship rolls, and the needle comes back out again. It goes in and comes straight out. I can't secure the stitch. In order to beat the ship's roll, I swiftly insert the needle through both sides of the wound, align the edges as best I can during one sideways roll, before the vessel briefly reaches its nadir and starts rolling back. The next stitch has to coincide with the next roll. I've never had less control of the needle. No scar? It is not going to be my best piece of embroidery. I pride myself on neat stitching. As a gynaecologist I introduced a comfortable (subcuticular) stitch cunningly buried under the skin to repair birth canal incisions and tears. It replaced the standard surface stitches to the most tender part of a woman's body, which many women complained felt like barbed wire.

Mandy is the perfect patient: stalwart when the stinging anaesthetic is injected; still as can be throughout the procedure; grateful at the end.

Coralie is an efficient and effective assistant. She cleans Mandy's neck and puts an invisible skin-coloured dressing over the wound.

'It should heal in about five days, because the face always has a good blood supply – as you can see...' I say, looking at her blood-stained skirt all the way to the hem. 'Keep it dry for forty-eight hours then come back to have it checked.'

'But I won't have a scar, will I?' Mandy pleads.

'I hope not,' I say. It's out of my hands now.

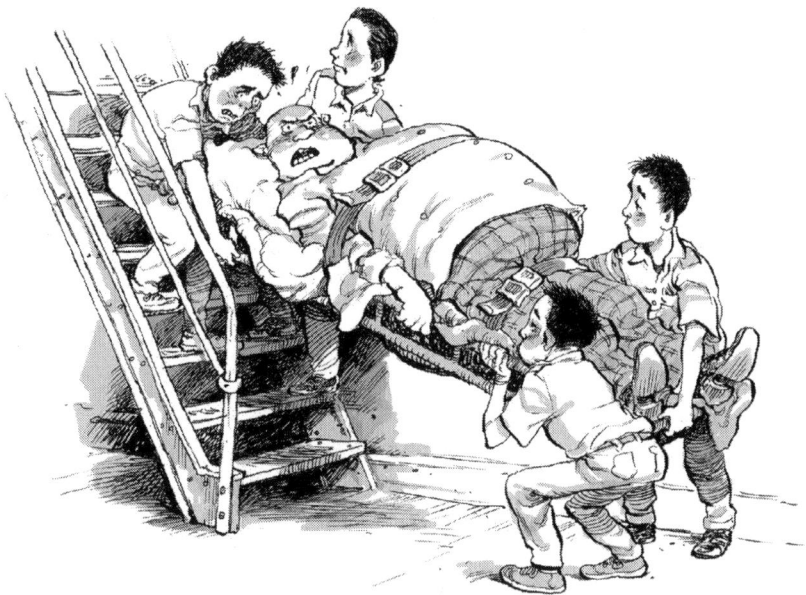

Days 12–15

Crossing the Line

Charles Darwin, sailing in H.M.S. Beagle in 1832, was forced to endure the age-old initiation ceremony of 'crossing-the-line'. He describes being *'placed on a plank, which could be easily tilted up into a large bath of water... lathered (on) my face and mouth with pitch and paint... and tilted into the water where two men ducked me. Most of the others were treated much worse... even the captain'.*

Sea Rainbow is about to cross the equator, at zero degrees latitude, thirty degrees west longitude. There will be three whole days at sea with no land in sight.

Some passengers are restless, bored and keen to arrive at Fortaleza in Brazil. Others are busy with crafts, art or drama groups, choir, dance lessons, lectures, bridge, deck games, socialising or solitary reading on loungers.

Tom has plenty of time to get on with his drawings on deck, trying to avoid giving medical opinions to passengers who trouble him with their ailments. In the afternoons he goes to the gym. He is looking annoyingly slim, fit and tanned, whilst I am paler, thinner and more stressed than when I boarded.

Coralie arrives for work on time, although she continues to ignore me as much as she can get away with.

Mr Richardson is in surgery with Vera.

'What sort of a night did you have?' I ask.

'Pretty good I think,' says Mr Richardson, looking at Vera.

'No. It wasn't. You were very restless,' says Vera, 'and you talked a lot in your sleep.'

'Did I? What did I say?'

'All rubbish. As usual.' Vera chuckles.

I check his temperature – 37.5°C, still up slightly, but improving. His oxygen saturation is ninety-five percent, at the lower end of normal. His chest examination remains unchanged. He is holding up.

I arrange to see him daily. There are *some* advantages to living with my patients.

Coralie, Liz and I are discharging gastros and there are no new cases at last. This includes Ron Sheehan. He is not, after all, 'a case'. And nor am I.

Each day I visit Rosa and each day the angry little blisters increase. Her skin is now maddeningly itchy. I prescribe a stronger antihistamine. She is fed up alone in the sunless inside cabin and misses her friends. All she can do is shower, sleep and watch TV. At least her chest is clear. She has spoken to her mother, who doesn't remember her having chickenpox as a child. So, she doesn't have a repeat infection due to any worrying immune deficiency such as HIV, just a natural lack of immunity to chickenpox.

Other crew members attend surgery dutifully to have their

insect bites, verrucas, ringworm, athlete's foot and acne checked, many of whom benefit from treatment. Some have neglected their conditions for months. Because of their full schedules, few find time to see the doctor. Despite it being highly infectious there are no more reported cases of chickenpox. Curious.

⚓

'Code Bravo, Code Bravo, Code Bravo, staircase B, deck two aft, starboard side. I repeat: staircase B, deck two aft, starboard side. This is an emergency drill for crew only. I repeat, this is an emergency drill for crew only.' It is ten-thirty a.m. on the second morning at sea. Ramon, the Safety Officer, is on the tannoy.

The eight-man emergency medical team run into the Medical Centre to collect the stretcher, medical bag with its equipment, drugs, suction and oxygen. It's a fire drill, so while the fire crews don heavy high-viz protective clothing and fire-fighting equipment, we prepare to receive imaginary cases of smoke inhalation and burns. Liz takes the two-way radio, communicating with the Bridge to report all medical personnel and stretcher team present, then receives instructions about where to collect 'casualties'.

I am relieved not to be leading the team. I don't know how to use the two-way radio for a start. No training. No certificate. I'd be lost trying to find 'staircase B, deck two aft, starboard side' in an emergency. With my sense of direction, I'd arrive just in time to witness neglected fatalities and view the ship's burnt-out hull taking in water.

Ramon has chosen one of the largest chefs as a 'casualty'. Below decks, he is stretched out on the corridor floor, the mound of his stomach lying on top of him. Liz and I ask him about injuries and burns, check his airway and breathing, and give him oxygen via a face mask, which one of the stretcher team produces from the equipment bag. The rest of the team roll the chef onto the stretcher with a lot of pushing and shoving, together with inevitable giggling. They set off down the corridor and start mounting staircase B. That's the plan. The chef is big and heavy, while the team of Filipino men are small and light. It is an effort to stop the chef sliding off the stretcher, despite body straps. There is a lot of grunting and shouting of instructions in Filipino. On the stairs the team slow down, trying to keep the stretcher level, but the men holding the top, bearing the heaviest load, are flagging. Suddenly one of the stretcher-bearer's knees buckles. He collapses, letting his side of the stretcher fall, pulling the rest of the team with him. As the chef tips sideways he hits his head on the stair edge, his arm slapping down onto the collapsed stretcher bearer's chest.

'Ow! You bloody idiot!' The chef shouts, his heavy face red to the neck.

'You too fat!' The struck stretcher bearer barks, clutching his chest, and catching his breath.

'Me? You're piss weak – that's your trouble – effing useless!' Chef holds the side of his head, which is starting to bleed.

'Now, *now*, *now*.' Liz raises her voice as she closes in on the scene. 'Come on. Calm down, everyone. Just hold still for a minute. Everyone be quiet.'

We check the chef's head. There is a small cut, bleeding energetically. A lump is expanding around it. There is no sign of injury to the stretcher bearer's chest, even though he is nursing it and groaning.

Liz applies a piece of folded gauze to the chef's cut, firmly held on by a bandage that passes under his chin. He adopts the dramatic stance of a real casualty now, holding his head and moaning. She radios Ramon to report the incident.

'Right, just make sure your patient is on the stretcher firmly, you boys,' Liz commands. 'Check your straps. OK? Are they tied securely this time? Let me see… Here. Make this one tighter. Now get a proper grip, all of you. Do you need any more hands?… No?… You're sure? Then when you're ready, give the signal and set off all together. Careful. Concentrate on what you're doing.'

Back at the Medical Centre we fill out an accident report while Coralie checks the casualty. She washes, glues and dresses his scalp wound, while he protests repeatedly about the fiasco. 'That's the last time I volunteer for any drill, I'm telling you,' I hear him say, '*last time*. Effing lunatics!'

'Put all the kit back, and then come and see me before you disappear,' Liz calls out to the stretcher team. 'Don't go.'

She tackles Ramon about the size of the chef over the two-way radio. 'Not what I would call sympathetic,' says Liz to no-one in particular. Turning to the stretcher team: 'I know it wasn't very fair for the drill, but don't forget that you might have someone that size – or even bigger – in a real-life situation. So, there'll be extra stretcher training here tomorrow morning at eleven.' The team grumbles. '*Listen*. Guys! I want you all back here at eleven. OK?' The men file out, returning to their regular jobs as waiters, deck-hands and lighting engineers.

A member of the entertainments team rushes in. 'We need some bandages and safety pins,' he says. 'Oh, and have you got any nappies?'

'What's happened now?' Liz asks.

'No. *Crossing-the-line*. It starts in two hours.'

'But listen. Can't you get old sheets from the laundry and tear them up? Bandages cost money. You'd be surprised how expensive they are,' Liz says.

'Well, what about two or three real life bandages at least? Haven't you got any cheap ones or used ones? And a few of those adult nappies or pads, whatever you call them. Oh, and eye patches – black ones.'

'Give him a couple of our old gauze bandages,' Coralie tells Liz. 'We never use them anyway. Don't know about safety pins. Wadja want them for?'

'Wouldn't you like to know?' He turns to me, grinning. 'You'll be there, won't you, Doc?'

I know all about the crossing-the-line ceremony from our family's five sea trips from England to Australia and back. We enjoyed joining in the hilarity then. Dad had been the 'barber' on one trip, delighting in lathering captives in foam and 'shaving' them, ready to appear before King Neptune to hear the 'charges' against them. Dad was a natural showman. But now the last thing I want is to be chased around the deck by whooping buccaneers, lathered in something disgusting, made to grovel in front of King Neptune, Queen Amphitrite dressed as a mermaid and all their 'court', then thrown fully uniformed into the pool in front of passengers and crew. No chance of maintaining a shred of dignity. I'm not about to ham a comedy act to amuse onlookers. And have I already mentioned the knickers?

Liz and the entertainments man disappear into the treatment room.

'I'll give Mr Richardson's antibiotic on my way to see Rosa,' I announce. That will keep me out of the path of marauding pirates.

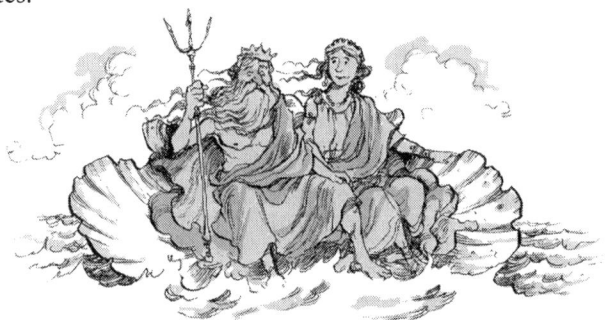

In the noon report Captain Strom again urges everyone to conserve water, even advising people to 'shower with a friend'.

Now that could lead to unforeseen public health consequences. He should have asked my advice first. For one thing, we are running low on condoms.

Mr Wayfield has stopped attending for inhalations. If he's better, is it due to the inhalations, the high doses of doctor and nurse, the passage of time, or witchcraft? This is the mystery of medicine. As Voltaire said, '*The art of medicine consists of amusing the patient while nature cures the disease.*'

Mandy's chin wound looks more ragged than I'd have liked as the edges knit together. Now it is up to the healing power of the good body.

Jesus returns for a review of his hand dermatitis. It has improved. 'Agent in Manila says I'm working in laundry. I want to work in laundry. I work in laundry in Pillipine. My contract says laundry but I wash up. I should be laundry.' So, this is the diagnosis – a contract dispute.

'You were supposed to be working in the laundry, not in the galley?'

'Yes, ma'am.' He sits with his hands on his knees, his shoulders heavy.

'Shall I have a word with the Chief Officer for you?'

'Yes, ma'am. Tell him I laundryman.' His face brightens up.

Later I ring Tallak's work desk in the Bridge office.

'Tallak, I've just seen a galley man called Jesus. He has hand dermatitis due to water coming over the top of his gloves. He's very unhappy, partly because of the dermatitis, but also because he tells me that he applied to work in the laundry and was told by the agent in Manila that that's where he'd be, but he's been put in the kitchen.' I use my authoritative voice.

'Yes. I know all about him. We didn't have any vacancies in the laundry so we've started him as a kitchen hand. If he gets on OK, he'll move to the laundry when there's a vacancy.'

'Does he know that?'

'I think so.' Tallak sounds vague.

'Is it alright if *I* tell him?'

'Sure. There should be a vacancy before he finishes his contract. Two laundrymen leave in about six weeks.'

'I'll let him know. Oh, by the way, why are we conserving water?' I slip into my hail-fellow-well-met voice.

'It was contaminated with oil in Cape Verde. The water was loaded from a tanker that must have been used for oil. By the way, that's confidential, you understand.'

⚓

There's more time to enjoy the ship's activities now that the noro outbreak is waning. Tom finds a table-tennis table, bats and balls in a side room, where he enjoys beating me at every game. He boasts that he will still win using only his (non-dominant) left hand. The ship's roll adds to the challenge of getting the ball back onto the table, accompanied by howls of delight or pique. One afternoon, during a match, Tom shouts, 'Look... *behind* you. A big splash and a tail! There's definitely something there. I saw a tail. Look! Over there. *There,*' he points. We stand, arms round each other, staring out of the window for a long time at the churning water rushing past, the white tops, curling waves and shadows of clouds far out, imagining glimpses of life. Nothing. I begin to wonder if there is anything living in the sea anymore. Has mankind unkindly fished the whole lot out? In the 1880s Robert Louis Stevenson wrote about the South Seas that '*a man might look overboard all day at... the many-coloured fish... sharks swarm there... to feast upon this plenty, and you would suppose that man had only to prepare his angle*'. By the end of the twentieth century, ninety percent of all the big fish in the sea had been taken.

We discover that a dozen table-tennis enthusiasts play

each other every afternoon, supervised by one of the lively entertainments crew, who keeps score.

On a few occasions we join in the passengers' games, until Tom admits that it doesn't look right when the doctor's husband repeatedly wins matches, especially as there are keyrings and pens as prizes. When he wins against Dick, the hitherto champion, and is presented with a bottle of bubbly, Tom feels particularly uncomfortable. Dick looks put out despite the handshake. After that we just play against each other.

Following Tom's success at knowing the tallest underwater mountain quiz answer, he starts to adopt a self-congratulatory air when the subject of quizzes arises. The printed quiz left on the lounge room tables in the mornings is an exception to this. It needs time, patience and concentration to attempt it. Alternatively, every evening for half an hour there is a popular quiz in the Pool Bar. Sometimes we arrive just as the questions and answers are being called out. Tom seems to know most of the answers, especially on the subjects of sports and entertainment. He's pretty good at the politics and history questions too. On the other hand, I am mainly competent at medical questions, unless it's a poor discriminator, like 'Which is the body's largest organ?' Is it the liver or the skin? It depends on the definition of 'organ'.

On the evening before arriving in Fortaleza, our table companions urge us to join them for the quiz. Derek, Pam, Mary and John are planning to commandeer a table with another couple of enthusiasts, Joyce and Len. Tom and I sit to one side, as the rules state that crew are not allowed to compete in passengers' games, and this contest is very public. There are fourteen tables of contestants, overseen by Cheryl, who wears bright pink lipstick and a matching evening dress with a plunging neckline. The quizzers call out, 'Come on, Cheryl, give us the questions.' 'Don't give us any of those wrong ones like last night.' 'Come on, Cheryl. Get going.' Cheryl smiles and hands out pencils and paper.

The theme for the night is Elvis Presley. Our table is confident, even Tom, despite him not being an Elvis fan. Question number two is, 'What was the first film Elvis appeared in, in 1956?' The table occupants bend towards each other and whisper suggestions – *Blue Hawaii*? Tom leans in and says in a low voice, 'If it was 1956, I reckon it must be *Love Me Tender.*'

'Are you sure?' says Len.

'Well, think about it. If it was '56… his first film… I'm pretty sure *Love Me Tender* was the first one,' Tom reiterates.

No-one else is certain so Mary puts down Love me tender in her neat, round handwriting.

Cheryl calls out, 'Question number five: Where did Elvis marry Priscilla?' Some of the questions seem so easy that there is a chorus of voices providing the answer, followed by 'shushes' to warn each other that surrounding tables can overhear. A loud false answer is then sent round the table to try to fool others into recording the wrong response: 'Graceland! Graceland!'

'Question number twenty: What was the cause of Elvis's death on the autopsy report?' I know this one. I mutter under my breath 'arrhythmia'. Tom tells the table. Mary can't spell it. I write it down on an old receipt from my pocket and slip it to Tom, who gives it to Mary. I remember the autopsy result because I can't for the life of me understand how an abnormal heart rhythm can possibly be detected at a post-mortem examination. It makes me wonder whether the real cause of Elvis's death was an excess of fried peanut butter and banana sandwiches. A form of hypercholesterol-sandwichitis.

Love Me Tender proves correct. Elvis married Priscilla in Las Vegas, where else? Arrhythmia is right. Our group wins. We whoop with delight. Then a man at the next table calls out, 'Hey! *They* can't win. The doctor's husband helped them. He gave the answers. Cheats! Invalid! Not allowed!' Other tables' occupants turn round and join in, booing and shouting for a recount to exclude our table. Cheryl looks nonplussed for a few seconds then calls out: 'Hello-o! Table eight! Has the doctor's husband helped with the answers?'

Everyone at our table looks sheepish. Mary says, 'Maybe one or two.'

'But if that's the case we can't allow you to win. Sorry guys. Against the rules,' Cheryl says, shaking her head and wagging the question sheet at us. She does a recount. The table with the hostile man wins, amid resentful mutterings from our table, which spills over into the aftermath, when Cheryl gathers up the pencils and answer sheets.

'Sorry,' she says, as she picks up ours, 'but they're the rules. I can't let it go when there's a complaint.'

'Oh well,' Derek says, to no-one in particular, 'we'll just have to be more subtle next time.'

'I don't think there will be a next time if there's going to be this aggravation. I can't believe people take it so seriously – all for a bottle of bubbly,' Tom says.

Len and Joyce rise to go.

'We weren't to know,' says Mary, standing up. 'Wait for us, we're coming to the show.'

'You coming?' Joyce asks us.

'We're staying to dance,' I say.

Tom and I move to seats close to the dancefloor and order glasses of prosecco to steady our nerves.

'*What a drama.* Who'd believe there'd be such a fuss? That's the last time I try and help out, clearly,' says Tom. He drains his flute in one gulp and orders another.

'Maybe the man on the next table thought that because you're the doctor's husband, you have access to the questions and answers through some sort of internal officer channel,' I say.

Tom smiles, but I can see that he is still piqued. 'Anyway, I've been meaning to tell you – I was on my way back to the cabin after the gym, just walking along the corridor in my shorts. This woman appears from her cabin – she must be late fifties, I'd say. She says, "Would you mind doing me up?" She stands in this dinner dress with the zip undone all the way down her back, you know, showing her bra straps, slip and everything. She says "Can you zip me up? I can't manage it." I say, "Sure" and zip her up. As I'm doing it – in the passage, hoping no-one sees me – I can see into her cabin. Would you believe it? She has this long rail thing rigged up all down one side. Well, I tell you, there must be thirty or forty dresses hanging from the rail. I couldn't believe it. She just said, "Thank you" and I walked on. She looked like Barbara – that one we saw with Reg, on deck. I'm sure it was Barbara.'

'*No!* So carnal knowledge in the corridor – eh?'

'They just can't help it, you know, when they see me in shorts...' We laugh as Tom downs his drink.

'I bet she's an all-rounder, with all those frocks. Point her out to me.'

'Have you got training or something tomorrow?'

'Lifeboat drill.' I pull a face.

'But you did it last week.'

'They're every fortnight. People will only remember if they practise time and again. Remember? When the Twin Towers came down, the only survivors from above the hundredth floor were made to do the escape drill by their safety officer once a month for years. They complained bitterly about the drills but they got out alive.'

'I remember. The Health and Safety rep went back in to check everyone was out and the tower collapsed on him. But what about tomorrow?'

'Do your run and come back for me at midday.'

Tom orders more prosecco.

The duo starts their set with *Wooden Heart*, one of Elvis's steady, slow jives from 1960. On the floor we shake off the small cares of the evening. Then it's *Jailhouse Rock*, from Elvis's 1957 film, a jive with terrific pace. We notice the shouty man from the quiz and his partner move onto the floor. We can't let *them* take over the jiving spotlight. It's a very fast jive. They struggle to keep up. We throw ourselves into the rhythm and give it fireworks. Clearly, we are the winners now.

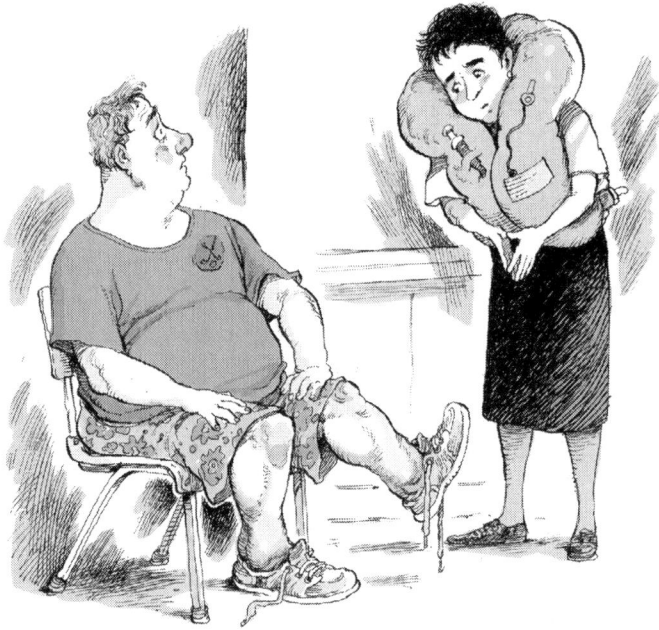

Day 16

Port Health

'Is an allergy!' Dr Fernandez declares, throwing his hand in the air.

Rosa stands with her pyjama top lifted to expose a clutch of pink spots on her abdomen. She looks embarrassed and seems to stare at me accusingly over Dr Fernandez's shoulder.

Tallak steps back into the corridor and closes the cabin door. 'So. Clearance?' he asks.

'Clearance,' confirms Dr Fernandez, nodding.

The five port health officials and I go our separate ways.

My bleep had gone off before breakfast. Tallak, the Chief Officer, asked me to go to the card room to meet Fortaleza's Port Health team. Dr Fernandez, in his crisply pressed white coat, had quizzed me in a heavy Portuguese accent over the green baize table.

When had it started? Had I done any diagnostic tests? Had she had it before? What were her symptoms? What treatment had I given? Any other cases?

Dr Fernandez, with his veined face and heavy grey moustache, had jotted down notes with nicotine-stained fingers. He'd looked at me gravely over the top of his glasses, which were perched on the end of his nose. I'd felt as though I was on a hard chair in a dim room with a bare lightbulb in my eyes.

Chickenpox represents a port health risk. Quarantine clearance had been delayed, resulting in passengers crowding around the gangplank complaining. Once Dr Fernandez decides to call it an allergy, Eric, the Cruise Director, makes the announcement: 'Passengers may now proceed ashore.'

The diagnosis is absolutely not an allergy. With small blisters? No way. Once you've seen chickenpox umpteen times it's a spot diagnosis. I am determined to keep Rosa in quarantine for the remainder of the seven days.

In the Medical Centre Mandy lays on the treatment room couch, while her friend from the dance troupe holds her hand. Liz is painstakingly removing the sutures from her chin with forceps and a stitch cutter.

'How's the wound?' I ask Liz, peering over her arm. Both Liz and Mandy say 'Good' simultaneously.

Moving round, I look at it more closely. 'You're a good healer, Mandy. Leave it to the air now, will you?'

'Shouldn't I wash it with Dettol, or put Germolene on it, or something?' asks Mandy, her speech distorted as she tries not to move her chin while Liz works on the last stitch.

'Not at all. The wound's closed, so germs can't get in now.

Just wash it when you're washing the rest of your face. It should be absolutely fine.'

Mandy's friend looks at the wound. 'It's really neat, Mandy. No-one will notice. Honestly, they won't.'

Mandy springs off the couch in her agile dancer's way. 'Let me see.' She goes over to the small round mirror on the wall and tips her head back. 'It's very pink.'

'That will fade in time, like all scars,' I say.

'Thanks so much, Doctor,' Mandy beams.

I am particularly relieved not to see a zig-zag, puckered line.

'I've still got gastros to discharge,' says Liz. 'I'll ring them now so they can get ashore.'

'Fine. I'll just get a coffee and a couple of biscuits. I'm famished.'

'There's three waiting. Notes are there. Mr Richardson's next.'

Biscuits gobbled and coffee gulped, I call Mr Richardson.

'How are you doing, young man?' He's on his own. A good sign.

'It's a few years since I've been called that,' he grins.

'You're looking better. How're you feeling?'

'More normal without that thing in my arm. I'm on the pill now.' He chuckles.

'Excellent. At least we know it's had fifty years of success. Let's have a look at you.'

His chest is clear for the first time. No fever, and his oxygen saturation is a healthy ninety-eight percent.

'Code Alpha, Code Alpha, Code Alpha. Deck seven forward, starboard side. Repeat, deck seven forward, starboard side.'

I poke my head round the door. 'Is that drill, Liz?'

'*No.* Don't know what it is. I'll run.'

'I'm coming… Mr Richardson, I have to rush – emergency. Come and see me in two days. Must dash, sorry.'

I speed up four flights to deck seven. As I arrive at the top, gasping, Liz is already helping a small woman into a wheelchair. Wheelchairs are kept on every deck. Passengers are standing around looking on. Our patient doesn't look at all moribund; in fact, she looks very well – sitting up, pink and talking. Why Code Alpha, a medical emergency?

As I arrive, I see that it is Alice. 'Alice? What's happened to you?' Her friend Pat stands close by.

'I don't know. I must have slipped on something and fell over,' Alice says. 'Silly really. I'm not hurt. Honestly. Just my ankle.' She holds it up, turns it and winces. 'It happened just like that. It's my fault. I was trying to be quick.'

'She just fell down,' adds Pat.

'No dizziness? No blackout? No numbness or weakness? No chest pain?'

'No, I don't think so. I just feel a bit shaken up.' Alice is holding tight on to the arms of the wheelchair.

'She's FAST negative,' Liz says, referring to the quick visual test for signs of a stroke: F-ace droop, A-rm weakness, S-peech impairment, and if necessary, T-ime to call an ambulance.

'Let's get you down to the Medical Centre to check you over properly, Alice,' I say.

'Can I come with her?' Pat asks.

'Oh, I'm causing such a lot of bother,' Alice sighs.

'No, you're not. We've got to be sure you're alright,' says Liz, pushing the wheelchair towards the lift. 'Let's go.'

Examination reveals that Alice has a fast irregular pulse, running at one hundred and fourteen beats per minute. Her ECG (electrocardiogram) confirms the condition: atrial fibrillation.

'You've got an irregular pulse, Alice, did you know that?'

'Oh yes, I've had it for years,' she says, waving her hand dismissively. 'I've been told the name, but I can never remember.'

'Atrial fibrillation?'

'Yes, that's the one. That's why I take warfarin, to thin my blood – oh, but you know all about it…'

'Nurse'll check your INR. Did you bring your yellow book?' It's an NHS shared-care booklet that patients carry to appointments recording their warfarin dosage, the recommended range of their INR blood-thinning test and their previous results.

'It's in the cabin. Maybe Pat could get it for me. Could you, Pat? It's in the top drawer of the desk thing, by the mirror. You know…' Pat takes Alice's keys and leaves. 'I didn't realise you can do that test here. I wish my GP would do it in her surgery. It'd save me a lot of time going up and down to the hospital. Honestly, it takes me half the day.' Alice clicks her tongue and shakes her head.

Alice's INR result is within the recommended range, but her ankle is swelling and bruising. Liz gives her two paracetamol tablets and applies an elasticated bandage. Alice flinches. Accident forms are laboriously completed for the Safety Officer, Ramon, and Alice is discharged back to her cabin.

I'm not at all convinced about her fall. Her heart rate was fast but she wasn't in heart failure. Her atrial fibrillation could have caused a tiny blood clot to sail off into her brain. Perhaps she'd had a transient ischaemic attack (mini-stroke), yet there was nothing to suggest it. I'd just have to bear it all in mind.

'They shouldn't use Code Alpha for someone who trips and falls, should they?' I grumble.

'They use it for all sorts. Actually, it's very rare that we get one that *is* serious, but obviously we have to dash just in case,' Liz says, clearing up.

'Shouldn't the crew be taught when to use Code Alpha – you know, the proper criteria for it?'

'They are, but actually it's difficult for them to be sure whether someone needs medical attention or not. Some of them don't have much education.'

Tom appears at the door. 'Hello Liz. Everything alright down here? Need any help?'

'Of course we're alright. Listen, everything's always under control in this department.'

'That's not what I've heard,' Tom teases.

'Well, the A team's on today, you see,' said Liz, putting on a superior voice, and pointing to herself and me.

'That'll explain it then,' said Tom. 'You two've got qualifications, I take it?'

'Cheeky beggar!' Liz exclaims.

'Take no notice of him,' I say.

'Oh, that's nice. No wonder my confidence is zero.' Tom turns to me. 'Have you got drill today?'

'Lifeboat drill. Remember?'

'So, I go ashore and be...'

The high-pitched general emergency alarm drowns Tom's voice.

I mime going to the cabin to grab my lifejacket.

As I return through the waiting area wearing the head-splitting fat orange vest with its reflective tapes, whistle and light, I see a patient sitting there.

'I'm sorry. It's crew drill. Can you come back this evening? Or is it urgent?'

'Nurse said for me to wait to see you,' says a stout man in green Bermuda shorts, a white cotton t-shirt sporting a golf-club logo, and unlaced deck shoes.

'Ah, in that case it'll have to be *very* quick. Come in, come in.'

Mr Gardner is in his sixties, worried about increasingly swollen ankles. He wants to go ashore but is struggling to fit into any of his footwear. I am surprised that he can see down to his feet. The tablets he shows me are for blood pressure, diabetes and cholesterol, ones he's taken for years.

As if in one of Charlie Chaplin's silent movies, I quickly examine him for the most obvious signs of heart failure, kidney disease and deep vein thrombosis.

'Have you put on weight this trip, Mr Gardner?' I speak fast, my voice raised.

'I haven't weighed myself, but I suppose my clothes are a little tighter.' He considers his words like someone with all the time in the world.

'Are you sticking to your diabetic diet?' He looks at me as if I've asked whether he's brought his own sandwiches for the voyage. 'Well, there *are* plenty of dishes for diabetics,' I add encouragingly – or, more likely, accusingly.

'Mm, I know,' he replies.

'Your blood pressure's high, you know – one hundred and seventy-five over ninety-five. Might be because of the weight gain. I'll add in a mild water pill. Try not to put on any more weight while you're on board, keep active and put your feet up whenever it's practical. See me in three days, or sooner if you're worried. Yes?' My spiel is rapid, sounding like a verbal warning about a building society investment. I am impatient, aware that I look like an orange humpty-dumpty and am expected elsewhere. 'Bring in a water sample as soon as you have time. I'm sorry, I have to go now,' I say, handing him a sample pot.

'Alright. But why have my legs swelled up like this?' He holds his legs out, staring at them. 'They're not like it at home.' Is this the time for an existential discussion on leg swelling?

I press my finger into his calf. It leaves the tell-tale finger-shaped depression.

'A build-up of fluid. Blood pressure, sitting around, and extra weight.' I unlock the pharmacy door, grab the tablets, stuff them into an envelope, scribble the instructions and thrust the packet at Mr Gardner. 'We'll sort the bill out later,' I say, shepherding him out of the door. Coralie would have approved. I finish the consultation in five minutes flat.

As I run up to the line of crew standing by my lifeboat, I call out, 'One-nine-two.' Everyone looks along the line, while I re-tie the trailing tapes of my lifejacket.

'I was just sending someone down for you,' says Alberto, our lifeboat team leader.

'Sorry,' I say. 'Emergency patient.'

'Bridge, Bridge, are you receiving me? Over.' Alberto, with his weather-beaten face, small crooked nose and dimpled chin holds the walkie-talkie close to his mouth. The reply sounds like a wasp trapped behind a window-pane. 'Lifeboat five – all crew present and correct. All crew present and correct. Over.'

⚓

At the debriefing, Captain Strom addresses me. 'Dr Taylor, you were late for drill.' How humiliating in front of all the Senior Officers. I wonder whether senior men find it easier to humiliate a senior woman than an equivalent man. Maybe there has been a study on it in the *Lancet,* or in the seafarer's magazine, *The Sea.*

'I had an emergency patient,' I say, thin-lipped, and stare him out with hooded eyes.

'Ah,' is all he says, then passes his attention to the Chief Engineer.

At least I am in the correct uniform.

There follows an exchange between the captain and Sergei about the repair of the lashing hook from the previous drill. Captain Strom tells Sergei to instruct the bosuns to check all the launching equipment and report back after two weeks. Sergei's gaze flicks to Anton, the Second Engineer, and their eyes lock momentarily. The Master has spoken.

———⚓———

I bolt my lunch while Tom chews his bean soup, bread and double butter. Our two-hour vacation in Fortaleza is about to begin.

'I love this,' I say, reading the guidebook while bumping along in the shuttle bus. 'The local Indians killed and ate the first Portuguese bishop and the first governor in the 1500s! *Serves them right*,' I hoot. 'They didn't realise they were going to set foot in the *only* part of Brazil occupied by cannibals!'

'That's not funny,' says Tom and we both laugh more loudly than is proper.

'Tell you what – sounds like a pretty turbulent start. Lots of massacres – of the Portuguese by the Dutch, the Dutch by the Portuguese, the Indians by both, the settlers' independence movement by the patriots and on and on. That'll be why they've got all these forts here.' Reading about the place brings it to life for me. Tom prefers to soak in the atmosphere and experience 'the feel' of it. Wandering about aimlessly, I call it. 'Anyway, what's the plan?' I gaze out of the window, but can only see tall blocks of unattractive new-build flats stretching along the entire shoreline behind wide yellow beaches to the distance.

'From what I saw, it's mainly a modern place. Not much historical stuff. The market started packing up by eleven-thirty. It'll be closed by now. Ah, yes, there's a pretty spectacular Art Nouveau theatre. No decent coffee shops though, but then I left late this morning and had to wait ages for the shuttle. There was a long queue for the omelette man. And you know, he won't beat the eggs, so it always ends up being a broken yolk with white round it.' We decide that he hasn't done the official omelette-making course and consequently won't be in possession of the certificate.

The blistering heat hits me as we climb down from the bus. The temperature must be over thirty degrees. 'Can we walk on the shady side, *please*?' I press my sun hat down low over my forehead, losing twenty IQ points in the process.

'Alright. *Alright.*' Tom is still not used to my irritable post-menopausal heat intolerance. Over the years my Newham patients had become familiar with me apologising for cold hands in August. Now I am more likely to brand them. The public don't realise that the real cause of global warming is the ever-increasing number of post-menopausal women in the world.

I look at the passers-by. We are in Brazil. I want to see local Indians, indigenous people, but the pedestrians all look European. It's just a colony. Where are the natives? Why hadn't they killed and eaten all the colonists as well as the bishop and the governor? It might have saved them from the tsunami of European diseases that slaughtered ninety percent of them.

The uneven pavements are lined with hawkers selling everything and nothing: peanuts, home-made sweetmeats, canned drinks, cigarette lighters, matches, small torches and keyrings. A kebab vendor looks indigenous with his strong stocky body, blue-black hair, smooth brown face, straight nose, and dark almond eyes. So, this is what he's come to. I wonder if his ancestors had eaten some of the bishop.

The rainbow-coloured stained glass of the Art Nouveau theatre is set in an extravagantly ornate cast-iron façade. It has delicate fan arches at ground level and a balustrade walkway along balconies on the first floor. Yet it is only a front, not part of the theatre itself. '*Very* South American,' I state.

'It was made in Glasgow and shipped in sections,' Tom says. 'Guidebook.' Passing under one of the arches we find a cool courtyard in the centre of which the actual theatre stands, as though it has been lowered in. No time for the tour.

Half a dozen city blocks away we find the Centro de Turismo. A stylishly converted nineteenth-century prison surrounding a sun-dappled quadrangle. A sign points upstairs to the 'Museu de Arte e Cultura Popular': the art gallery. Instead of glass panes, the window openings are covered in a lattice of green wood framing the bright sunlight through its triangular gaps like diamond lozenges and allowing a blessed breeze in. Three skinny tortoiseshell cats lay in the yard below under a tree drooping with ripe mangoes. Outside the courtyard gate, market stalls display t-shirts, dolls in traditional costume, lacework and the fridge magnets of tourist paraphernalia.

I turn back to look at a carved head in the gallery. The size of a grapefruit, in taupe-coloured stone, the flat face with its broad nose has a serious, mournful look, resembling a generic human ancestor. I want to possess it, to cradle it in my hands and take it home, to protect it from what is to come. The future.

Suddenly Tom shouts, 'Here's our bus! We're *going*.'

'But what about the stalls? This won't be the last bus,' I plead.

'No time. *C'mon*. Look, it's *three* o'clock. We've got to be on board by half past. *Come on*. Why've you always got to push the limit?' Tom runs down the broad wooden stairs. I dawdle behind.

Inside the bus, Liz and Lee are seated close together halfway down, hand in hand.

I greet them. 'What did you think of Fortaleza?'

'Not much actually,' Liz says, making a face. 'But it's the place for hammocks. We got one in the market.' She shifts the large bag on her lap. 'That's all,' she says, rounding off the conversation.

'Are they an item?' Tom asks, as we sit three rows back.

'I don't know. It's not a subject of discussion. I suppose they must be, but then we saw Liz with that receptionist in Tenerif-eh. Remember?'

Near the bus stop on the quay, crew sit on the ground

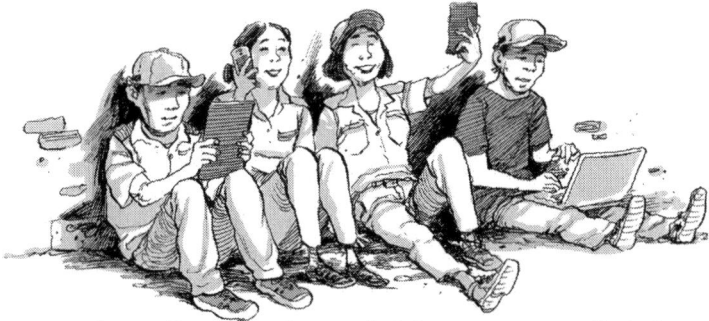

against the walls of the Seamen's Mission, caps pulled down shading their eyes, making last minute connections to families in Manila, Mumbai and Mauritius. They don't look up. The sacrifice of their being at sea for eight months at a stretch, away from children, spouses, parents and siblings, tugs at me. Some spend years at sea. Some, all their working lives. The Seamen's Mission provides free transport, internet and support.

An Anglican priest, John Ashley, was standing on the shore of the Bristol Channel in 1835, when his son asked him how the hundreds of men on passing ships managed to attend church. It prompted Ashley to establish the Seaman's Mission. The ministries spread and are now in fifty countries. Seafarers welcome the free communications, refreshments, leisure activities, transport, spiritual and practical assistance. A God-send.

⚓

Back in uniform I dash into the Medical Centre, grab a crew return-to-work form and run upstairs to Rosa's cabin. Ron Sheehan is limping down the stairs on the other side of the central handrail.

'Woah, Doc, another emergency?'

I'm out of breath. 'No – I just like people to think I'm terribly busy.' Grinning, we pass on.

Rosa comes to the door in rumpled pink pyjamas, her face puffy from lying down too much. She looks forlorn and doesn't smile.

'I'm sorry about this morning,' I say, stepping into the dim cabin.

'Who was vat man?' She puts on the light.

'The port health doctor.' I sit down in the only chair by the dressing table.

'He says I hab allergy, not ve uvver ving.'

'He only said you had an allergy because he didn't want the whole ship to be quarantined – so that passengers could go ashore. Anyway, how are you?'

'I better. When can I go to my friends and my cabin? I sad here. No light six days.'

'I know. It's been miserable for you. Let's see your spots.'

Rosa reveals scabs and scars in different stages of healing. 'See vis? Here. *Bery* itchy,' Rosa says, scratching a group of scabs on her left hip.

'In fact, they look fine, Rosa. Really. They're healing nicely. But try not to scratch. It'll make them more itchy. Anyway, you can be discharged tomorrow. Go back to your cabin in the morning, then you can go to work. Give this form to your manager.'

'*Oh?*' Her face lights up, then she curtseys. 'Thank you, Doc, I so happy.' She curtseys again. 'Thank you. *Thank you.* I can go, now?' She starts to gather up her clothes.

'Not *now*, Rosa. *Tomorrow* morning.'

'Oh, tomorrow… OK. Thank you, Doc. I so happy.'

I hear the scraping sound of the gangplank being winched in and feel the engines rev up with their seismic rumble.

In the Medical Centre Liz is phoning the gastros. 'Only three left,' she says, punching the air with her clenched fist as she puts down the phone. 'Should all be out by *tomorrow*.'

'Tomorrow! Thank goodness for that. Maybe we'll have some peace at last.'

The phone rings. Liz answers. 'Listen. Bring her down in a wheelchair now.' She puts down the phone. 'There's a passenger with breathing difficulties coming down from the Pool Bar.'

Two minutes later a bartender arrives with Pat in a wheelchair, accompanied by a companion. Pat is struggling to breathe.

'I'll take her, thanks,' says Liz, wheeling our patient swiftly into the resuscitation ward. She throws a backward glance at her friend. 'Would you mind sitting in the waiting area?'

'Will she be alright?' the friend calls out, frowning.

'Don't worry. We'll look after her.' Then Liz addresses our wheezing passenger. 'What's your name, dear?'

'Pat,' she puffs out the word in a short musical breath.

'I remember, you were with Alice the other day, weren't you? Listen Pat, can you get out of the wheelchair and onto the bed?' Liz asks.

'Yes... I think... so.' Pat moves slowly, grunting with each expired breath. Liz helps her onto the high hospital bed and takes off her deck shoes.

'Tell me what's happened, Pat,' I say. Her breathing sings in a strangled way. She has a swollen, blotchy face.

'I don't know,' she wheezes. 'I must be allergic... but I don't know what to... I've had it before... last time it was prawns... but I haven't had prawns...' She pauses for breath after every few words.

I listen to her chest. High-pitched wheezes in all areas. The air is squeezing in and out of swollen breathing tubes, sounding like bagpipes.

Liz takes her vital signs. 'BP ninety over sixty. Pulse one hundred and four, oxygen sats ninety-three percent.' She fits an oxygen mask over Pat's face, turns up the oxygen and lays her down on the bed.

'I can't... breathe... *can't breathe*. Let me... *sit up*,' Pat says, her face panicky, frightened, sweating.

Liz raises the back of the bed and helps her off with her t-shirt.

'Better?'

'Yes,' Pat whispers.

Liz puts a surgical gown on Pat, who grunts with the effort of struggling into the sleeves.

'It certainly is an allergy. Don't worry. We'll sort you out,' I say, my heart hammering. 'Give me adrenaline one in a thousand, hydrocortisone two hundred and chlorphenamine ten.' Liz is already at the resuscitation trolley pulling out syringes, needles and ampoules. 'You're not allergic to any medication are you, Pat?'

'Not... that I... know... of.'

'Are you taking any medication?'

'No.'

She is concentrating on the effort of breathing.

Liz and I check the drugs. I look at the clock. Five fifteen.

'This is adrenaline. It'll make you feel a bit strange but it'll help the breathing. Sharp jab.' I inject it into Pat's upper arm.

Liz is putting an intravenous line into her other arm. I move round to the line and start injecting the antihistamine, then the hydrocortisone slowly. 'I'm giving you antihistamine and steroids. The antihistamine helps the itching and swelling, and the steroid calms everything down – though it takes a little while to kick in.'

I watch Pat's face while Liz takes another set of observations. 'Pulse one hundred and twelve, BP one hundred over sixty-five, sats ninety-five,' Liz says. Pat's brown hair is matted with perspiration.

'Put up a litre of normal saline,' I say, then, looking at Pat, 'How are you feeling?'

'Don't know... odd... itchy.' Pat is still breathing hard. Red wheals are breaking out on her arms. 'Can I... have... water?'

'Can you swallow alright?' I ask.

'I think... I think... so.'

Liz fetches water, lifts the oxygen mask and Pat drinks. Her Adam's apple moves up and down. Good. No significant problem with throat swelling.

Liz collects a bag of saline from one of the banks of cupboards around the ward walls and connects it to Pat's IV line. She checks the flow. 'What rate?'

'A litre over two hours, then review,' I say.

'I don't have to... be here for... two hours... do I?' Pat gasps.

'Probably not. I expect you'll be better before then, but we'll just have to see how you go.' I stand close to Pat, watching for signs of improvement.

'I'll give the registration form to your friend to fill in. OK?' says Liz, moving towards the door.

'She won't know much. Only met on board.' Pat calls after her, using one breath per sentence.

I look at the clock. Five twenty-five. It is more than five minutes since I gave adrenaline.

'How's your breathing now, Pat?' I observe her chest movements, trying to judge whether her breathing is visibly improving. An end-of-the-bed-o-gram.

'I think it's a bit easier.' Is she saying what she thinks I want to hear?

'Big breath.' Through the stethoscope her chest sounds like a barrel organ.

I fetch another ampoule of adrenaline as Liz reappears.

'I'm giving another adrenaline one in a thousand.' We check the ampoule. 'It'll take a while for the other drugs to work,' I announce. I don't say 'up to two hours'.

Liz records the adrenaline dose and the time given with the other observations on a hand towel on the bedside table.

The second shot of adrenaline goes deep into Pat's well-toned, bronzed upper arm.

Ideally, according to my expensive resuscitation training, we need to keep her under observation for six hours, but with our limited team it isn't practical, and probably not necessary considering we live with our patients.

'Is Coralie here?' I ask Liz.

'I've called her. Should be in soon.' We glance at each other.

'She can keep an eye on Pat while we get on with surgery.'

'I'm sorry to cause... such a nuisance, Doctor,' Pat says.

'It's *fine*,' I say, 'we just don't want to let you go until we're sure you've recovered. You'll stay with us for a while at least. We can order something from room service.'

'I'm not hungry.'

'Pulse one hundred and fourteen, BP one hundred and ten over seventy, sats ninety-eight percent,' says Liz.

'The adrenaline is making your pulse race but you're improving. Oxygen level is better. On the mend,' I tell Pat, as my heart slows towards normal. 'Quarter-hourly obs, don't you think, Liz?'

'Sure... Your friend can come in now, Pat. I'll give her a call,' says Liz.

Pat closes her eyes, resting her head back.

Coralie turns up. She looks older, her face somehow collapsed in on itself.

I leave Liz to give Coralie a handover while I return to my Lilliputian office to start surgery. Bracing myself for complaints, I go out to the waiting area. 'Sorry to keep you all waiting. We've had an emergency to deal with.' One woman says, 'I'm first sitting. Is there time for you to see me?'

I get a move on.

Finishing surgery with a sense of urgency, I go next door to check how Pat is faring. Pat's friend is sitting holding her hand. 'Hello, Alice. It's good of you to stay,' I say.

'I'm not Alice, I'm Barbara.'

'Of course. Sorry, Barbara.' So, *this* is Barbara. The Barbara heavily petted by Reg in the deck shadows. The 'zip-me-up-in-the-corridor' Barbara.

Normally I have an extremely good memory, except for names and people's occupations and where they live. It's a kind of brain-syndrome-thing. Medical matters I remember well, and grievances.

'How does she look to you?' I ask Barbara.

'She's looking more herself now,' Barbara says. 'She did frighten me when she said she couldn't breathe. It happened so *fast.*'

Barbara is in her late fifties, plump and shapely, with very fine permed hair dyed auburn, the sort that she wouldn't be able 'to do a thing with' once the perm grows out. She is wearing the remnants of today's cosmetics.

I turn to Pat. 'How are you feeling?'

'Much better thanks, Doc. I think I must have slept. But what was *that* all about?' She levers herself upright.

'Let's see. When you're allergic to something you've eaten or drunk you usually react within about an hour. Are you suspicious of anything you had within an hour of it all starting?'

She purses her lips. 'Not really. The last thing I drank must have been a couple of cocktails on deck at the sail-away party. I think it was rum punch, sort of an orangey colour, delicious. Oh, *don't tell me* I'm allergic to cocktails – that would be just too cruel.'

'Well, you could be allergic to one of the food colourings – maybe orange, one of those E-numbers. A food dye. Red, orange and yellow cause the most reactions. Ask the barman what went into the punch… What are Pat's obs, Coralie?'

'Stable,' says Coralie, showing me the observations chart with readings transferred from the emergency paper towel. 'The IV's about three-quarters through.' She is in her element. Like throwing a switch, Coralie's response to medical emergencies is prompt and competent.

'Let's see your rash, Pat.'

She pulls up the sleeve of the blue check surgical gown. There are faint pinkish-brown shadows where the angry red wheals had been.

'Right. I think we can let you go, provided you behave yourself. No more orange cocktails.'

'I'll stick to the green ones.' Pat grins, shifting her legs over the side of the bed.

I give Pat instructions in case of a repeat reaction, supply her with antihistamines and discharge her.

⚓

'I didn't think much of *this* place,' says Reginald at the dinner table. 'All my-eye-and-Betty-Martin. Did anyone else take the Hop-On Hop-Off bus? I had the same trouble you did, Derek, in… where was it? Madeira?'

Reginald never addresses the women at the table. It is as though they are invisible.

'I suppose you hopped off and couldn't hop back on,' says Derek.

'Yes, a blooming swindle for eleven pounds.'

'We didn't take the bus. We decided to wander, but in fact it was a bad idea,' Derek says.

'It was your idea. I wanted to go on the city tour.' Pam looks peeved.

'It was fully booked,' Derek says.

'Yes, but we could have gone on the reserve list. There are always people who drop out.' Pam isn't going to be easily mollified.

'There aren't always. Anyway, we did go to the market. It had a lot of stuff we wouldn't see at home – fresh peanuts, your actual brazil nuts... ah, and there were great big sacks of brown powder at one stall with the name 'Viagra' written on a piece of cardboard. God only knows what was in it. We didn't buy any. I mean, there was no price on it for starters.'

'We booked the city tour before we came,' Mary says for the benefit of Derek and Pam. 'The guide said that the native people are only half a percent of the population now.'

'Amerindians,' John adds.

'Apparently there were millions of them when the Portuguese arrived, but they died of disease or were killed, so they were. The rest have mixed in with all the other folk – Portuguese and coloured people,' Mary says.

'Same in Australia, and North America,' Tom says. 'The Aborigines were deliberately killed by the colonists. There were Aborigine hunts in Australia and poisonings,' Tom looks at me. 'Ruth knows all about it. She lived there.'

'I think the last state-sponsored massacre was in 1921.'

'As late as *that*,' says Mary, shaking her head.

'In Tasmania too,' Tom urges me on.

'Yes. The police and troops swept the island from end to end in the 1800s, catching and killing as many Aboriginals as they could. The last full blood, Truganini, died in about 1880.'

Mary tuts. Our waiters arrive with steak, schnitzel and pork chops, and our table-mates scrutinise their plates of food, waiting to start eating together.

'Talking of which – did you see in the *Sea Rainbow Times* there are big bushfires in Australia?' Reginald says.

'They happen every year,' I say. 'It's actually vital for the ecology, for renewal of the vegetation.'

'No, but this is around Canberra. That's the capital, isn't it? Hundreds of homes burnt out and people have died. A right rum-do.'

'Ruth has family in Canberra,' Tom says, looking at me with concern.

'Yes, my dad's partner, Saint Jean, and her family live there. I'll have to e-mail them and see if they're OK. I didn't know…' Saint Jean is the nickname we gave to Dad's adorable long-suffering partner. He isn't an easy man to live with.

'Och, but did ye see the dolphins this evening?' Mary asks.

'We got a video of them,' Pam says.

'*No.* What time?' I ask, forgetting about family possibly dying in bushfires in Canberra.

'Five…' Mary starts to say. 'Aye, I'd say five-thirty. We'd not long left port. Dozens of them. All leaping up. Marvellous.'

Derek says, 'Maybe you were busy seeing the Code Alpha lady.'

'Mm,' I murmur, allowing myself the tiniest of nods. 'We're looking forward to Salvador. It sounds like it's got a lot more going for it than Fortaleza.'

'It was the first capital *and* a big slave port,' says Derek.

'My great-great-grandfather, or was it great-great-great… well, he was a slave bought by the British Army in 1800 – for the West Indian Regiment. The government bought thousands of slaves to be soldiers,' says Pam. Everyone looks at Pam.

'Of course, they were used in the Caribbean, to keep order. Africans took to the heat better than British soldiers.' Tom knows his history. 'There were over two million slaves there – in the Caribbean. And I can tell you that Britain had the biggest slaving port in Europe: Liverpool.'

'How did you find out about your ancestor?' I ask Pam.

'I got my DNA done, didn't I, Derek? I was shocked when it showed five percent West African. So, I started to research it. None of my family knew. It caused quite a stir, I can tell you. I had to go to the National Archives in Richmond, then the Army Museum, in… er… Chelsea, and I got his discharge papers. Archie Padgett, he was called. It was quite emotional really.' Pam stops speaking and pokes her pork chop.

—⚓—

As Tom and I approach the bar, I can see Ron Sheehan just inside the entrance.

I hiss, 'That man there – he's the Arsenal fan.'

'The first one? Yes, I've met him before,' says Tom.

Ron is perched on a bar stool next to another man. They always seem to occupy this station together in the evening. Ron is upending a bottle of beer, topping up his glass. Both men have their eyes glued to a football match on the TV.

'Did you get our result?' Tom asks Ron. In Arsenal-ese it means they've won.

'Yes, nice one – four nil away. Not bad. Makes the two points we dropped to Liverpool even more irritating.'

'Come on. Look on the bright side – United've got a couple of nasty games coming up.'

'I know,' says Ron, taking a slurp of beer, 'but this not knowing what's going on till it's already happened is wreaking havoc with my nerves.'

'Steady on, Ron, you don't want to have a seizure on board with the doctor's prices.'

'The doctor'll give me a discount. I'm a favourite of hers,' Ron says, nodding towards me. 'It's alright for you though – you're getting off in Rio. You'll be jumping up and down at Highbury while I'm stuck here getting the news second-hand.'

'Whatever happens, Ron, be comforted knowing I'll be thinking of you as the goals go in.'

They laugh in a hollow way.

None of the usual faces are in the Pool Bar. It seems that everyone has headed for the Ocean Lounge, attracted by the night's entertainment. I've never heard of the cabaret singer, Baron Wild, but that doesn't mean he's not famous. Doing medicine means missing out on a lot of popular culture. Then there is the fact that the ship is starting to roll, so those with delicate stomachs will have taken to their cabins.

Dave is just starting to sing *Love Sick Blues*, made famous by Hank Williams in 1948. Despite my protests that it is a hackneyed old country and western piece, we step onto the floor. We dance an even-tempoed jive, which puts us in a good mood. We're on our own. Carrie and Dave nod and half-smile to us. We lurch with the ship's movement, Tom shouting '*whoa*', laughing and hanging on to my arms. I had been an amateur gymnast until my early twenties, specialising in the beam and high-low bars, so pride myself on good balance. We find ourselves skidding involuntarily down one end of the floor, then sliding along to the other end. It is the last song of the set. Lee takes over and we motion to Carrie and Dave to sit with us.

Tom offers drinks.

Dave orders a half of draft.

'Just a tonic with ice and lemon, thanks. The voice…' Carrie points to her throat. She has a clear, smooth complexion, sparse makeup, and hair pulled back from her face. She is wearing a pale blue cat-suit. Close up she looks about forty. I don't know why I am surprised to see that she has three piercings in each ear.

Tom waves to the drinks' waitress. Petite with jet black hair cut in a neat bob, her round face and dark button eyes make her look too young to be working, too young to be out late. She puts down four bar mats then writes Tom's order on a pad with her child-sized fingers.

'We like seeing you dance. It always makes our effort feel worthwhile. Nice to get a response,' Dave smiles.

'Isn't it quiet in here tonight?' I say.

'I think they've all gone to bed after trailing round Fortaleza all day,' says Dave. 'It wasn't very stimulating. I hear one of the women, who's usually here, wasn't well either.' How does news travel so fast? 'Is she alright?'

It is a recurring ethical dilemma.

'She should be alright,' I say.

'You've had a busy trip? Some sick people,' Dave says.

'It seems to be settling down now. Thank goodness.'

'Have you played guitar for long?' Tom asks Dave, rescuing me.

'About twenty-five years. Started in my teens. Taught myself.'

'It's very good. Reminds me of Jeff Beck.'

'*Jeff Beck*? He's my hero. Really, it would be *great* if I sounded like Jeff Beck. I listened to him a lot when I was learning. He's *the best*. The Yardbirds – with Eric Clapton and Jimmy Page – you remember?' Dave leans forward, elbow on the table.

'Yes, terrific guitarists. I've always been interested in Wes Montgomery and Jim Hall too,' Tom continues.

'Wes Montgomery was an *icon*. Jazz guitar started with *him*. But then Jim Hall was cool. Lovely touch, smooth jazz.'

The doll-like waitress arrives with our tray of drinks. She expertly sets them on their mats while the ship rolls.

'To my mind you can't beat Jimmy Reed for the blues though. Goes right through you. Bit like a male Billie Holiday,' Tom adds.

Carrie and I look at each other with sympathy.

'I was going to say that most of the early jazz musicians died young – drink, drugs, car accidents, you name it.' Tom knows that the only guitar music I like is classical or flamenco. 'Did you two get on in Southampton?'

'Yes, we've been on for four months,' Carrie says crossing her eyes. 'We were only supposed to do two, but the next group let the company down so we're doing extra.' She sips her tonic. 'To be honest, it's a bit of a strain after a while. I know we shouldn't complain, being on a cruise ship, seeing the world. But the cabin gets smaller as the trip goes on. It's like some sort of "through the looking glass" experience, and then the whole thing starts to feel very repetitive. We won't be sorry to finish. Are you on all the way round?'

'Only to Rio. Tell you what – that will be enough for me, too. It's been *so* busy. Not the least bit what I expected,' I say.

'The last doctor had some pretty tricky cases too,' Carrie says.

'So I understand.' I didn't want to pursue the subject of dead bodies.

'Where are you from?' Tom asks.

'King's Lynn,' says Dave.

'My brother lives in King's Lynn. He teaches drama and English at Springhill Secondary,' I say.

'We haven't got children,' says Carrie. 'We couldn't have, with our way of life. We're hardly ever home. We can't even keep a cat, let alone children.'

Carrie doesn't look upset. She is matter-of-fact. Dave looks relaxed.

Lee is playing *C'mon Everybody*, a favourite fast jive. My toes are tapping. 'Come on, Tom, let's do this one.'

'It's too fast for you,' Tom teases.

'For *you*, you mean.'

Tom takes his jacket off. In fast tempo we are pushed up and down the floor by the sea's swell.

'Keep your arm tight – *tight*,' Tom commands as we wobble and stagger.

'I *am*. If only I had a *strong lead*.'

'Well, don't *you* lead then.'

'Someone's got to.' I stiffen my elbow and push hard against Tom's hand.

It becomes more and more difficult to keep to the beat *and* maintain balance. Even for a gymnast. We flop back down in our seats, panting.

'She just can't keep up the pace,' Tom announces between breaths. 'This is what happens when you're married to an older woman.'

'Or when your husband's too doddery to stand upright,' I jibe.

Carrie smiles. 'Not quite the weather for it.'

We lurch down to the cabin.

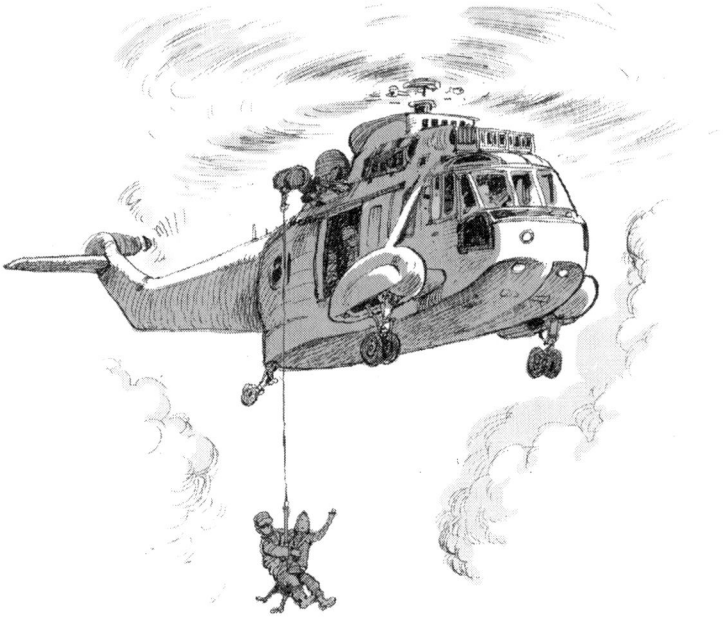

Day 17

Mr Marquez

'Good morning, ladies and gentlemen. Today is Sunday the nineteenth of January and we have just docked in Salvador, Brazil. The weather is fine and sunny with a predicted top temperature of twenty-six degrees and a light breeze. I have been informed by the Port Authorities that *Sea Rainbow* has been given clearance, so passengers may now proceed ashore. I am pleased to announce that there are no longer water restrictions on board. I repeat, water restrictions have been lifted and passengers may drink water from the cabin taps after ten a.m. this morning.' With a flourish, Eric, the Cruise Director, completes his announcement. 'There is also no need to *share a shower*. I wish you all a very pleasant stay in the wonderful town of Salvador.'

At six a.m. the grinding and clanking noises start as the ship prepares to dock. Tom is sleeping on his good right ear with his congenitally deaf left ear uppermost. There are some advantages to having one deaf ear.

I brush my hair and eyebrows with the spiky plastic hairbrush that sets my neurones firing and slip into uniform. Stepping over the high sill onto the deck, I drink in the clean, bright air as it pats my face with its cotton wool touch. Among the few passengers on deck, one is studiously doing her power-walking laps – five to a mile – head down, her brow wrinkling when someone crosses her path. She wears one of those unattractive khaki sun hats with an insufficient brim so beloved of the English. I walk behind her to the bow of the ship where I can lean over the rail and see the deck-hands, supervised by a Junior Officer I don't recognise holding a two-way radio to his ear. Three deck crew are struggling with the heavy metal mooring line, or hawse, feeding it out over the side through the hawsehole. It has a three-metre length of thin rope attached to the end, which looks far too insubstantial to hold any boat, let alone one weighing 35,000 tons. When the ship is within six metres of the quayside the hawse is thrown ashore to one of the local dock workers, who braces himself and expertly catches the narrow rope, pulling the massive metal hawse towards him so that, with the help of a fellow docker, they loop the weighty metal lasso over a bollard. Of course, they couldn't possibly catch the huge steel hawse itself. It would take their hands off. The ship would crash against the quay and blood would splatter all over its clean, white sides.

Salvador is built into the side of a steep brown cliff, revealing rows of brightly coloured two-storey houses, the lower buildings stacked up from near the water's edge to the cliff's halfway point, clearly separated from the upper section of large official-looking mansions around the summit. There is an immensely tall, cream-coloured shaft from bottom to top, which houses a lift. In a large glass-windowed cabin at the top, I fancy I can make out faces. Above the cliff small lazy clouds wander across a piercing blue sky.

'Hello.' A woman in her seventies with a sun-crinkled face and old-fashioned blue-rimmed glasses is at my side. 'You're the dancing doctor, aren't you? I've seen you and your husband up in the bar. Are you dance teachers?'

'Heavens, *no*. We just like dancing,' says Dr Modesty-Herself.

Dance teachers? She can't have any idea that dance instructors, like my teacher, John, the East End Fred Astaire from Dennis Drew's Dance Studio in Upton Park, knew every toe, every heel, every drag, tap and angle of the foot, turn of the head, position of the arm and lean of the body in every dance, both for the men's steps and the women's in ballroom, Latin, jive and sequence dancing. Like the London taxi drivers' knowledge, a veritable PhD. And light – so light. No pushing. My feet just glided where John led.

'It must be nice for you to have time on deck. You've been *so busy*, haven't you?' she says, her hand on the rail next to mine.

'Mm. It's the first time I've been out here to watch the ship docking. I love to see a new place loom up and come into view for the very first time. It's exciting.'

'Yes, it really is, but you saw the dolphins, didn't you? Or were they porpoises? I can never tell. Round the other side, towards the back. Must have been about thirty of them. Jumping right out of the water, like that.' She gestures their leaping motion.

'No! What time was that?' I take my hand off the rail and face her accusingly.

'Only about fifteen, twenty minutes ago.'

'No! I missed them. That's *really* annoying. I wish the captain would announce when there's wildlife, then we could all see it. I'll have to speak to him. I'll call him down to my office and have Words.'

She chuckles. 'The passengers wouldn't appreciate being woken up at this time of the morning. Besides, if everyone hung over the side, the boat would capsize.'

'But we've all done lifeboat drill. It'd be good practice.'

We both laugh. Such a wonderful idea – this whole trip-thing.

The dining room smells of bacon and toast. I pass Pam and Derek at a two-person table, empty cereal bowls to one side, tucking into Full Englishes, the centre piece a large rack of toast. We exchange brief greetings. I can see exactly why they've brought a larger set of clothes for the end of the cruise. End of the cruise. This is it. Today's port, then Rio, then home.

I am surprised at the wave of relief I feel. I am *so* tired. Drained. I just want it all to end. As a junior doctor working one hundred and twenty hours per week, I had looked down the stairwell at Leicester Royal Infirmary where I trained in general surgery wondering whether I should jump just to escape the exhaustion.

However, the thought of returning to my busy East End practice suddenly presents a manageable workload, a relaxed way of life in comparison to being on call 24-7, not even enjoying a single Sunday morning to lie in and recharge the batteries.

It reminds me of the Jewish joke in which Moishe goes to the Rabbi to complain about the lack of space and privacy in his cramped flat with his wife and five children. The Rabbi persuades him to take in successively chickens, a sheep, a goat, a dog and a cat. Moishe's complaints escalate, so the Rabbi instructs him to remove the animals. Moishe is ecstatic. 'I can't thank you enough, Rabbi. Such a lot of room we have! And so quiet!'

Tom pokes his head round the surgery door. 'Hello darling. Have you got drill or training today?'

I swivel round in my chair. 'No, nothing as far as I can see.' I normally only call Tom 'darling' when I want to emphasise a point in an argument.

'Good. Meet me at eleven on the quayside.'

'Right-o.'

Mr Gardner is back with his swollen legs.

'How are they?' I ask, looking down at his feet in their Velcro-fastened grey sandals.

'Maybe a bit better, but not a lot.'

'Did you pass more water after you started the water tablet?'

'I don't think so. I'm not sure. I always pass a lot of water anyway. My doctor says it's because of my diabetes.'

'Right.' I'm not getting anywhere. 'Let's see what the pressure's doing.' I tighten the largest blood pressure cuff around his ample upper arm. 'One hundred and sixty-five over... ninety-two. A bit better, certainly not worse.' Statistically speaking it has not changed, within the margins of error of the machine and the operator. I press my finger into his swollen foot. It leaves an impression. I repeat the process up his leg until no more impressions form. That is at his lower calf, just above the ankle. Better than three days ago. Possibly. I am persuading myself.

'I'll do your blood sugar.' I don't want to ask Coralie, who knows how to work the machine. She isn't speaking to me again.

The finger prick doesn't bleed. I stick the lancet in deeper. Mr Gardner flinches. Now I have a good drop of blood. It splashes onto the end of the testing stick and onto my notes. I put the stick in the machine, then mop my notes with a tissue. 'ERR' appears on the visual display. I glare at it.

'I think it's the other end,' says Mr Gardner.

'Yes,' I say. There is a pictorial guide to the use of the machine inside the open lid of the box. I run my eyes across it, hoping Mr Gardner can't tell that I am learning how it works. Every brand of machine functions differently.

The lanced site hasn't congealed yet, so I squeeze out another drop of blood, drip it onto the opposite end of a new testing stick and insert it into the machine. 'Ten point seven,' I announce.

'Yes, but that's because I've just had breakfast about three quarters of an hour ago, so it's bound to be up now, isn't it?' Mr Gardner is appealing to my reason. (In non-diabetics, the upper end of normal after food is 7.8 mmol/L.)

'Well, the idea is for your tablets to control high sugar levels *after* meals. Was it your normal breakfast, like you have at home?'

'No, here I have a cooked breakfast after my porridge. I might as well, as I've paid for it. At home I just have porridge.'

'That'll explain it then. If you're going to have a bigger breakfast on board, you'll need to take extra tablets to keep your sugar down. Take an extra one with your breakfast from now on. We've got your tablets in stock, so you can order more if you're running out. At any rate you've only a few days left to go.'

'We're all-rounders. One hundred and two days.'

The Chief Engineer appears. 'Are you busy?' Sergei must be six foot four. With his dark unruly hair, heavy black eyebrows, square jaw and perpetual five o'clock shadow, he can appear intimidating. A bit like the Incredible Hulk or the Terminator. How does he even fit into a ship's bunk? It crosses my mind that he might suffer from an excess of growth hormone – a condition called gigantism. Should I do a blood test?

'Did you want to see me?' I feel suddenly vulnerable, cricking my neck to look up at him.

'Yes, I can come in?' He looms.

'Do. Sit down…' I put my head round the door and ask Coralie for Sergei's notes. Sergei looks less menacing sitting down, but he still seems to fill the room.

'It's my back. I got slipped disc three years ago and it gives me pain and it's sometimes numb down this leg.' He puts his hand on his left thigh, runs it down to his calf, then rests it on his knee. 'My doctor in Russia did lot of tests and I had exercise treatment, but still it comes and goes. I come just for painkillers. I'm nearly run out.'

'Let me have a look at you. Can you get up on the couch?'

Lifting each leg to test his knee reflexes takes all my strength. How can one leg weigh so much? The examination reveals an absent left knee reflex, to be expected after a slipped disc, but his back and leg movements are surprisingly full. There is no apparent pain when he moves, nor loss of sensation in the affected leg. I notice he has huge hands. Maybe they are just in keeping with his stature. He climbs off the couch easily.

I look at Sergei's record. There are repeated entries for one hundred co-codamol tablets, a mixture of paracetamol and codeine. He is prescribed the strongest version.

'How many tablets do you take a day?' I ask casually.

'I don't know. It depends. Between four and six maybe, more if I have more pain.' He sounds irritable at being asked.

'Every day?'

'Yes.'

'Do you have any days when there's no pain, or the pain is less?'

'I can't say about no pain. It's a bit different each day.' Now he is staring me out.

'Did you know these tablets can be addictive?'

'Addictive? No. Nobody said.'

I bet they did.

'Yes. Codeine is related to morphine, so it can lead to addiction.'

'Are you saying I'm an addict? I only take the tablets when I need to.' He starts to sound threatening. He is between me and the door.

'No. I'm just saying that you have to be careful. On the days when you have less pain, can you manage with fewer tablets, or without?' I am determined to keep the conversation as low-key as possible.

'I never tried.'

'What about your posture and your workstation? Are they good for your back? Are they OK?'

'Yes. I'm sure. The physical treatment nurse – what do you call her?'

'Physiotherapist?'

'She told me how to stand and sit and I have a good chair in the office.' He straightens his back. I straighten mine.

'And a firm, comfortable mattress?'

'Not so much.' He looks away and blows a sigh through compressed lips, impatient to finish.

'Do you get morning pain?'

'Some mornings.'

'Can you requisition a better mattress? A firm one – like an orthopaedic mattress.'

'I could, but I have to have a letter.'

'OK. I can do that. Who shall I make it out to?'

'Hotel Manager – Oleg.'

'In the meantime, I want you to start cutting down on the co-codamol. We can do it gradually. We don't want you to get addicted,' I say, recruiting him to an imaginary joint agreement. 'I'll give you something else to take instead and we'll work down slowly,' I say as though we've definitely agreed a contract.

'So, how many tablets are you giving me?' He frowns,

deepening his hollowed eyes, which look ready for combat. I feel like prey.

'Let's work it out.' I take a piece of paper. 'These are the days… so – Wednesday, Thursday, Friday six tablets, then Saturday, Sunday, Monday five, then four, four, four etcetera. Come down by one tablet every three days, until you get to one. After three days of one you can take either half daily or one on alternate days for three days, then stop. That will take just over three weeks. I'll give you anti-inflammatory pills to take twice a day as well, if you need them.'

'So, I'll only get sixty-five tablets.' Being an engineer, maths is his subject.

'Yes, but you'll have the other tablets, which aren't addictive.' I can see strife ahead for the next doctor, who'll curse me.

'But will it work? What if it doesn't work?'

'It certainly *should* work. But if you're in trouble, come down – we always have other options. We can move you on to the milder strength of co-codamol if necessary. We're here every day.'

'O-K,' he says slowly.

'*Fine.*' I say cheerfully, as a psychological ploy. 'Good,' I emphasise, and stand up to indicate the consultation is over.

'What about my letter?'

'You can pick it up this evening, or in the morning.' As he goes out, I note his loose-limbed walk. No stiff, back-protective gait.

Detective Inspector Taylor writes 'CAUTION. OVERUSING CO-CODAMOL' in bold.

Coralie has seen two crew members, one for a repeat prescription of the pill, the other to collect free condoms for shore-leave.

Marion, manager of the ship's boutique, is next. Tall, very slender, in a thin multicoloured dress and high heels, with dark hair pulled back severely from a pale, bespectacled face. At the back end of her thirties, she looks tired.

'I keep on getting this pain in my right side. Like a stitch, but it comes and goes. Sometimes it makes me feel sick.' She pushes her knuckles into her lower abdomen with her right hand and screws up her face.

'How long has it been there?'

'Since the beginning of the trip. I thought it would go away, but it's got worse – it comes more often now.'

'Had it before?'

'No. Could it be trapped wind?'

'Well, we'll see. I'll have a look in a minute. Anything seem to bring it on or make it better?'

'Paracetamol helps for a short while, but then it comes back. Rennies don't do a thing. If I lean against the counter that can set it off. Sometimes it goes down the inside of my leg.'

'Periods OK? Any discharge? Any new sexual partners?'

'My periods aren't on time but they never have been. My next one is about due, I think. No new partner. I've been with my same one for a year.'

'What about contraception?'

'We've always used condoms.'

'Every time? Ever miss?'

'Hardly ever miss. Not recently anyway.'

'OK. So, take your knicks off and hop up,' I say, drawing the curtain round the couch.

Doing the internal, I detect a lump in her right ovary. It's tender to pressure.

'Aah! There. Yes, that's where it is. Yes, there!' Marion jumps.

'There is a bit of a swelling on that right ovary.' 'A bit' being my attempt to minimise the impact of the news. 'Are you up to date with your smears?'

'I had one last year. A swelling on my ovary? What does *that* mean?'

'Well, the most common cause is a cyst, like a water blister – usually quite harmless, but a nuisance. If it's a cyst, it normally goes down on its own after about three periods. But you'll need a scan to check properly, in more detail. Rio will be the place for that as we're there for three days. Will that be OK?'

'Yes. What do I have to do?' Marion wrinkles her brow, her lips slightly apart.

'I'll do the referral and nurse will let you know the arrangements. Cabin number?'

'Two-one-eight. You don't know what it is then?'

'Don't worry about it right now. We'll get the information back after your scan – though the result will probably go to the new doctor by then.'

'Won't you be here?'

'I disembark in Rio.'

'Oh, I wanted you to deal with it.'

'Most of the "dealing with it" will be over by the time the scan comes back. It'll just be a matter of confirming the diagnosis and deciding if anything more needs to be done.'

An ovarian lump is always a worry. I reflect on whether I should arrange a Ca 125 blood test, a marker specifically for ovarian cancer. How do I explain to Marion that the Ca 125 is advisable without raising her anxiety even more? But then she's probably already thought about the possibility of cancer. Any patient told of an internal lump naturally tends to think of cancer. Having the cancer blood test could reassure her that every stone is being turned. But what about ectopic pregnancy? She said she was using condoms. With a twenty-five percent failure rate over twelve months and Marion waiting for her period to come, I kick myself for not doing a pregnancy test. Damn.

I type the scan request for the hospital and ask for the report to be sent to the Medical Centre, then e-mail the Rio port agent, copying it to Uncle Tom Cobley and all, as per the protocol.

Collecting a urine bottle for the pregnancy test and a sheet of headed paper in case I need to leave a message under Marion's door about getting the blood test, I rush off.

Didn't we say eleven? *On the quay?*

I wait, hands on hips, assailed by the smell of cigarette smoke drifting across the quayside from crew members and passengers outside the port terminal. People stroll by, some going ashore, others already returning.

Mr Armsure and Harold approach with carrier bags, Harold trailing a few paces behind Alfred, complaining, 'I told you we wouldn't get fresh milk 'ere. They breed *beef* cattle. I *said*. Milk doesn't hold in this weather. It's all sterilised. I *told* you, but you wouldn't listen...'

'Oh, 'ello Doc. You orright?'

'Yes thanks, Mr Armsure. Waiting for the husband.'

'Are yer, lass? Very good. If we see 'im, we'll tell 'im.' They passed by. 'Yes, but still we got them brigadiers...'

'Why you want more food, Alf, beats me ...' They bicker on up the gangplank, their voices carrying out to sea.

Eleven-thirty a.m. I walk over to the terminal and look in through the entrance to the stalls and small local shops.

Tom is sitting on a bench with Ron, their heads bowed, deep in conversation. As I approach, I can see Ron showing Tom his mobile phone. 'Maybe Chelsea will do us a favour next week...' An Arsenal post-mortem.

'We didn't say meet inside *the terminal*,' I snap as I plant myself in front of them. 'I've been waiting on the quayside like a right lemon. We said *on the quay at eleven*.'

Ron gets up. 'That's me off. Leave you to enjoy your day.' He walks to the exit and lights a cigarette.

'Why you *always* have to get it wrong I don't know,' I carry on, so cross at losing one-quarter of my holiday that I allow myself the sour pleasure of being unreasonable.

'Alright, don't *go on* about it. Where do you want to go?'

'Into town, of course. Anything to see?'

'We have to go up in the lift.' Tom waves his hand in the direction of the buff column.

The lift leads out onto a cobbled street lined with a palette of pretty pink, blue and yellow colonial buildings. A cute, pure white church draws me over to a large glazed recess within the church wall. Behind the glass window, as if in a lounge-room display cabinet, a metal object catches my eye. Made of iron, it is in the shape of a mouth with a ligature attached to the corners. The upper 'bit' holds a small central rounded spike pointing downwards. The item is called a 'scold's bridle'. As a punishment it was fitted into the mouths of female slaves, especially those who were too talkative or insolent. I stare at it for a long time. If Mr Tenerif-eh had deigned to give one of his port talks about our slave trade route, I might have been forewarned. According to the description, five million African slaves were imported to Brazil between the 1500s and the 1800s. They worked on sugar plantations, in cattle-ranching, agriculture, mining and domestic service. The account went on. Salvador was the first port to receive slaves in the Americas because of the short sea crossing from West Africa, assisted by Atlantic currents. Life expectancy was little more than twenty years. Fifty percent of the children died before the age of one. And yet more. There are branding irons. I mean to leave but feel rooted to the spot, torn between not wanting to know another thing and wanting to know everything.

Propped up at the back of the alcove sits an actual photograph of slaves in regimental rows working on a plantation. A copy of a painting by Jean-Baptiste Debret shows a trussed male on the ground being whipped by his owner. Slaves comprised half of the population. The country didn't even ban slavery until 1888. I feel as if I am descending back down the lift shaft. I turn away. Compose my face. Search for Tom.

———⚓———

In the restaurant our waiter brings us home-made iced limeade.

'Are you studying here at the cookery school?' I ask him.

'Yes. Second year.' His English is perfect.

'How many years do you do?'

'Just one more year, but I want to be a chef, so then I'll have to find a position.'

'Are you from here?' asks Tom.

'I come from Fera de Santana. Do you know it?'

'No, we've just arrived on the cruise ship,' I say.

'Americans?'

'From England, London. Have you heard of London?' It's a joke Tom likes to repeat.

'My cousin lives there. Wilson? Willsden? I don't remember.'

'Your family's been in Brazil a long time?'

'Long time,' he raises his hand. 'My great-great-grandparents were slaves from Angola, worked the cotton plantations, but our family have lived in Brazil all the time after that.'

'What about your new president, Lula?' Tom wants to know.

'I think he'll be great. He'll help the people. Anything will be better than the military. Excuse me.'

He attends to two customers who are standing inside the doorway.

'Mm, this looks alright. I'm glad I found it,' says Tom, looking round at the room's dark wood panelling and hot buffet. Ceiling fans whisk the steamy air.

Volcanic, bubbling tubs contain eye-wateringly spicy fish, veal and pork stews, some with kidney beans, another of Tom's addictions. Hell-red sauces stand threateningly along the back edge of the buffet. Prawns make up half a dozen dishes.

'They should be left in the sea. Poor little grubs,' is my one-woman prawn protest. 'Fancy a huge animal like you eating bucket-loads of pupae the size of your little thumbnail. Leave them to their natural predators.' I could easily have carried a banner and marched, if I'd known where to protest.

'I *am* their natural predator,' says Tom, as he helps himself to a large bowlful.

Talk about taking a set of bigger clothes on the voyage. We demolish our feast as though we haven't eaten for days. Being fed three full meals daily is becoming a habit. Eating begets appetite. A mountain of cloying, creamy desserts on a huge Vesuvian cake-stand beckons. And Pam-like, I try 'a little of each', to Tom's 'I see you've given up on your figure then.'

Letting our banquet settle, we sip coffees while I eye an accompanying plate of small brown sweetmeats.

'Sweetened condensed milk and butter, heated until it's thick like toffee, cooled and rolled in chocolate. It's a famous Bahian sweet – brigadeiros,' explains our waiter.

'Yum. All part of a well-balanced diet.' To prove it I eat all four, one after the other. The sugar rush will accelerate me down the hill to the ship.

We step into the street, dazzled by the brilliant sunlight. The ship's map leads us along the main tourist thoroughfare lined by art shops. Tom is interested in the abstract paintings. I am drawn to the still lifes. One whole and two cut avocados sit on a small blue table, the used knife lying beside them. The insides of the avocados glow a ripe, luminous golden-green, ready to scoop out and eat.

'I *love* that one. Shall we get it?' I say. Tom is bound to agree to avocados.

'Where are we going to put it?'

I don't know if Tom is referring to the luggage, or to our well-covered walls at home. I suspect that our two weighty cases won't even comply with the generous marine allowance of thirty-two kilos each, let alone the prospect of trying to squeeze in a painting. I acquiesce. Something about that painting stays with me still.

Clouds loom and the breeze refreshes our skin.

'We have to head back,' Tom says, checking his watch.

'No, wait! Down there. There's music! Let's just see.'

Tom groans.

A band of musicians is playing near the end of the street outside a blue and yellow-striped baroque church. The musician's instruments are strange: a long bow with a single string, a tall drum, a kind of metal cone struck with a switch, and a notched length of bamboo that, when rubbed, sounds like a stick dragged along railings. The tambourine is the only familiar item. Two young male dancers somersault on the pavement and throw high kicks at each other, never making contact. Their dark perspiring bodies glisten. The lined face of the singer is impassive, his song more of a monotonal chant in a rasping voice like Rod Stewart's. The beat dictates the dancers' jumps, while a small crowd stand around clapping.

'It's Capoeira,' I say. 'Slaves weren't allowed to fight so they started the dance as a sort of martial art. From Angola, or maybe from London.' There was a Capoeira club two streets away from us in Hackney.

'*Come on*,' hisses Tom. 'You always have to be late!' He grasps my wrist.

―⚓―

The gangplank has already been loosened, ready to swing in to the side of the ship and collapsed for storage.

'*Doctor Taylor*. Did you get lost?' says the security officer.

The funnels emit two sonorous booms.

—⚓—

Messageries Maritime *Caledonien,* Sydney to Marseille, 1967.

En route from Australia to Marseille on a French half-cargo ship, I had been ashore with my best friend, Janey, and two French conscript soldiers on their way home to France. Dawdling as usual, we arrived back at the ship fifteen minutes late. To our horror both soldiers were thrown in prison, 'in the brig'. There they remained for a whole week until the ship docked in Marseille. They were treated badly, with a wooden bench to sleep on, one blanket each and only potato and bread for rations. Janey and I would sneak down to the brig in the rocking bow of the ship to take them treats. Crew took cigarettes, first-class passengers took cake and brandy.

This time Maritime Law is on my side.

In 1629 a charter was passed stating that all ships sailing from British ports were obliged to carry a surgeon on board. In 2006 the Maritime Labour Convention confirmed that 'a ship's doctor must be carried on any ship with 100 or more persons on an international voyage of 72 hours duration or longer'.

The ship had to wait for me.

—⚓—

On my desk is a urine sample from Marion. The pregnancy test is negative. Phew.

Shore referrals for crew are expensive for the company. I check that I've obtained the go-ahead from Dr Wallis, put the respective referral letters in envelopes and write up the medical report for the ship's end-of-cruise log.

Rio in two days. We are due to leave the ship and fly home the day after our arrival. We have a whole day to look around Rio before the next doctor arrives.

Coralie hasn't turned up. Someone presses the bell in the waiting area.

I call in a tall, heavy man whose hairy ears stick out, accompanied by his small, thin wife in a loose blue sun dress and sensible buff sandals.

Mr Marquez speaks with a slight Portuguese accent. 'I have dizziness. I thought I was going to drop down. And sweating. I sweated like a pig. It was today... about three o'clock.'

'He was nearly a grey colour. Very pale,' Mrs Marquez adds in a quiet voice. Mr Marquez glares at her.

'What were you doing?' I ask.

'Nothing. I just finished playing shuffle-board. Good game. I won.'

'No palpitations or chest pains, numbness or tingling?'

'No. I had it before – but not as bad as this. I had to lie down. If I hadn't, for sure I would have fallen, I'm telling you.' He looked too squat and solid to fall over.

'How long did it last?'

'About five minutes, I think. Yes, maybe five or ten minutes. About that.'

I look at him. He has a ruddy face topped by a shock of black hair peppered with grey. In his eyes there is a fatty arc partway around the iris. His nose, which looks as though it has once been broken, meets a thin upper lip. At sixty-five he appears strong, even combative, as though he's been a boxer.

'Does your doctor know about the dizzy spells?'

'Yes. She did all the tests and I had one of those... what's it called? *Ana*?' Mr Marquez demands of his wife.

'It was a, what you call it in English? *Eletrocardiograma*,' he says.

'Electrocardiogram,' I confirm.

'Yes, yes. But one for all the day and night,' explains Ana.

'The results were all good,' says Mr Marquez, looking at Ana as though she's criticised him. 'Nothing bad to find.'

'I see. Well, let me check you over.' Coralie's familiar noises start in the office next door.

As predicted, Mr Marquez's lying and standing blood pressure, pulse, ears, carotid arteries, chest, heart and abdominal examinations are all within normal limits.

'Can you pass a sample of urine?'

'I've just been. If you give me water I will go later.'

I open my door. 'Coralie, can you give Mr Marquez a glass of water and a urine pot, then do an ECG and blood sugar please?'

I look at the previous end-of-cruise medical report. It provides all the statistics: the number of noro cases, flu, repatriations, accidents, hospitalisations and significant medical conditions. I check our online noro log – forty-seven cases, fifty-three if I include 'observations'.

'Here.' Coralie puts the results down on my desk. Mr Marquez's ECG, blood sugar and urine test are all normal.

'Come in.' I beckon the Marquezes. 'I can't tell you why you've had this dizzy spell. All your results are normal – the same as with your GP. All I can say is to take it easy and let's see how you go on.'

'Do you want to see me again?'

'Only if you're worried about something.'

'OK. Come on, Ana.' I don't like him. Can't put my finger on it.

Coralie comes in.

'There's a deck-hand here with arc eyes. I've irrigated them but you need to see him for the accident report.'

She hands me his notes.

Anjan is nursing his right eye with a wet gauze swab,

blinking with his left, which is bloodshot. He sits down in a dirt-streaked boiler-suit, an oily rag hanging from one pocket and his protective goggles from the other.

'What happened?'

'I'm welding a pipe in the engine room. A small place. No room. I take off the goggles. Welder flashed my eyes. Too much pain.' His face shows it.

'Let me see.' He takes the swab away from his right eye, but screws it up against the overhead light. I switch off the light.

Examining each eye in turn with the ophthalmoscope reveals constricted pupils and inflamed conjunctivae (the white of the eye). Putting anaesthetic then fluorescent drops into his eyes makes him blink but shows that there are no corneal ulcers.

'Where are you from, Anjan?'

'Nepal, ma'am.'

'Can you read English letters?'

'Yes, ma'am.' I am grateful. I don't have a chart in Nepali script, and even if I had, I wouldn't have known which of the curly Nepalese letters he was reading. They all resemble wriggling stick insects suspended from a washing line.

I hold up the eye chart. 'Cover your right eye. Read from the top.' I point. 'A – D – F – H – Zee – P – T – Ix.' He hesitates. 'Ver...'

'Double-u,' I give him.

'... Erhh...'

He stops midway along the fourth line using his left eye, along the third line with his right eye. I don't know anything about arc eye. I've never come across it. His vision is more affected than I expect, assuming his vision was perfect previously.

We work through the accident form together.

'This goes to the Safety Officer. One moment. Stay here.'

I nip out to the nurses' office.

'What do I give for arc eye?' I ask Coralie under my breath.

'Eye pad and painkillers. It'll be better in a coupladays.'

'Have you got any painkillers in your cabin?' I ask Anjan.

'No ma'am.'

'Nurse will give you an eye patch to rest your right eye and some painkillers. You can take two tablets every four hours and I'll see you tomorrow. You'll be off duty until then. Let your manager know and give him this sick note.'

'My eye – I'm worry for seeing.' He looks anxious.

'Don't worry. Your eyes will be better in a couple of days.'

'But I can't see.'

'Don't worry, Anjan. It *will* get better. Go and see nurse for the tablets.'

———⚓———

Over artichoke salad Mary talks about the churches on the walking tour. 'I felt worn out after number six,' she says, shaking her head. 'So elaborate; lots of white, blue and gold and too many fiddly bits, so there were.'

It is Jim who mentions the church's role in slavery. Everyone around the table seems to know more than Mr Tenerif-eh ever imparted.

'You know, when the slaves escaped from protestant owners, the catholic church insisted on them being baptised and then freed them,' Jim says.

'More like a recruitment drive if you ask me,' Derek adds with a chuckle.

Pam points out that the slaves were meant to be brought into the church as equal 'brothers in Christ', yet their descendants occupied the bottom rung in San Salvador, so what went wrong? She explained about Candomblé, a mix of Catholicism and African beliefs. 'They hid images of their own gods inside figures of saints. People will always find a way when they're denied their culture.'

In true Reginald style, our man had sampled the local liqueur, cachaça, made from sugar cane, the most profitable export from the plantations in slave times.

As I sit listening to the conversation, it makes me think of what I'd learned from my East End patients: that people who initially appear colourless and lacking in personality turn technicolour once their lives are revealed. The more I know of a patient, the more interesting and memorable they become.

I am reminded of a woman who called for a visit twice a week from her sofa complaining of backache and a persistent cough. We GPs would wrangle over whose turn it was to visit her in her smoke-filled front room, until I decided to go weekly and find out about her life. She had been a neglected child in a large chaotic Mediterranean family and was given too much responsibility at too young an age. A failed marriage took over her adulthood, producing three children who, now grown, agitated the GP surgery. 'Somebody's got to do something.' Our growing rapport didn't cure her backache or cough, but she called less. I became 'her doctor' and she 'my patient'. We had an understanding and a mutual respect.

Tom and I link arms as we walk past the gaming tables and saunter into the Pool Bar. The pool, just outside the double doors, has been drained for the end of this section of the cruise and deck-hands in white overalls are covering the blue pit with a huge tarpaulin. We settle into our seats while Lee plays *Moondance* by Van Morrison, a lovely slow jive.

Dave and Carrie are at a rear table having an argument. Dave is looking down, hands fidgeting under the table. Carrie is staring hard at him, with pursed lips, saying something I can't hear. No eye contact.

'See that woman over there in the cream blouse?' Tom draws my attention.

'Where?' I look around.

'Don't stare. See the man in the blue shirt?' says Tom in a hushed gossipy tone. '*There*, just to the right of him – the woman in the cream blouse.' Tom points.

'Don't point. Next to Alice?'

'She's the one who asked me to zip up her dress in the corridor.'

'Yes, it's Barbara, one of Alice and Pat's friends. Was she really the one with Reg that night – the-groping-on-the-deck business?'

'Yes. It was *her*. She has a whole rack of dresses all along one side of her cabin. Must be about thirty or forty of them.'

'I know, you told me… Come on. Let's do this one.' I take Tom's hand.

'It's just about to finish,' Tom resists.

'Never mind…' I pull at him.

The loudspeaker crackles: 'Code Alpha, Code Alpha, Code Alpha, cabin four-five-two, starboard side, repeat cabin four-five-two, starboard side.'

I run. Down. Down again. Along. Odd numbers. Other side. Along again. In through the open door.

Mr Marquez is lying on the floor, his shirt undone. Ana stands off, grim-faced, staring.

Coralie is performing chest compressions.

The stretcher team unpack equipment. Lorenz puts the automatic defibrillator next to Mr Marquez's lifeless body.

On my knees, I say, 'Stop compressions.'

Putting my ear to his mouth, I feel the artery in his neck. No breath. No pulse.

I squeeze his nostrils and blow into his mouth, slowly, twice. My heart is banging.

'Restart compressions.'

Switching on the machine, I attach the defibrillator pads to his chest.

'Stop compressions.'

The machine gives orders in a Stephen Hawking voice. '*Analysing rhythm... Shock advised... Everyone stand clear.*'

'Stand clear!' I bark, sweeping my gaze round the body to ensure no-one other than Mr Marquez will be electrocuted.

'*Push shock button,*' Stephen says.

'Shocking!' I press the button.

The body jumps.

'Resume compressions,' I call out over the machine's voice: '*Shock delivered.*'

'I'll take over,' I tell Coralie. Exhaustion sets in after two minutes of performing chest compressions and Coralie is puffing and sweating, red-faced. I smell a whiff of alcohol as my head nearly collides with hers. I pump down hard on Mr Marquez's chest. 'Secure the airway,' I pant at Coralie.

Lorenz passes Coralie a nasal airway tube. She deftly lubricates and slides it into Mr Marquez's left nostril, attaching a self-inflating oxygen bag, which she squeezes rhythmically.

Two minutes.

'Rhythm check,' I exhale, my arms aching.

'*Analysing rhythm,*' Stephen agrees. It sounds odd that the machine instructs us.

I stare at the ECG. It is normal. Slow, but *normal*. My heart slows.

I feel for Mr Marquez's carotid artery and his groin pulse.

'*Pulse check,*' Stephen commands. A bit late.

'I can feel a pulse,' I say, amazed. There is a faint groan. It is Ana.

'He's breathing,' Coralie announces. I breathe in deeply.

'Blood pressure?' I asked rhetorically, attaching the blood pressure cuff. 'Eighty over fifty. That will have to do. Right, let's get him down to the Medical Centre.'

The stretcher team unfurl the stretcher. They gather up equipment, working quickly and silently.

I stand up, suddenly aware of stiff, aching knees. For the first time I notice the Chief Officer, the Hotel Manager, the Safety Officer and the Security Officer all standing in a semi-circle looking on. What are all these men doing here? Is it a last chance to see the knickers? A short bespectacled man stands just by the open door, looking in. I remember him from the crowd gathered at Alice's fall on deck. What is *he* doing here?

In the Medical Centre Liz starts the paperwork, recording the details as she follows Coralie and me into the hospital.

Coralie puts up an intravenous line, takes blood and commences IV fluids. Mr Marquez is unconscious. He is attached to an ECG monitor and receives oxygen via nasal tubes. I insert a urinary catheter into his bladder. He doesn't stir. Completely unconscious. Ana isn't with him.

Liz records his vital signs, which look surprisingly normal, but he hasn't regained consciousness, barely responding to my knuckles pressing on his breastbone to assess a pain response. I've never looked after a post-arrest patient. Why hasn't he woken up? Will he ever wake up? Is he brain-damaged?

'Anything else we need to do?' I ask Coralie.

'Blood sugar.'

'Of course.'

I look at Mr Marquez's ECG tracing. No sign of a heart attack. I compare it with the one we'd taken earlier in the day. No major change. So, I assume that he's suffered from a rhythm disorder that has gone on long enough to stop his heart – like Elvis. Lucky me; and lucky Mr Marquez. A rhythm disorder is the best diagnosis for getting any heart restarted quickly. As most cardiac arrests are due to heart attacks, barely ten percent of patients survive out-of-hospital resuscitation.

Mr Marquez groans loudly. 'Mr Marquez? *Mr Marquez*? Can

you hear me? It's doctor. You're in the Medical Centre. Hello! Open your eyes. *Can you hear me?*'

Hearing is the first sense to return. No response. Another loud groan. It is as though he is in pain. Like a wounded animal. What from? Bruising to his chest? Muscle pain from the electric shock? Headache from the chemicals released after a cardiac arrest? S.M. Search Me. In hospital these patients are transferred to an intensive care unit, where a whole experienced team of intensivists look after them. I have to get him off the ship to a proper hospital where they know what they are doing and have the staff and equipment.

'BM's nine point eight,' Coralie calls out.

It's an acceptable blood sugar under the circumstances.

Ana appears. Another howl roars out of her husband.

'Why does he do that?' she asks.

'He must be in pain. He's not awake,' I say. 'We'll give him something for it.'

The intravenous morphine works a treat. Mr Marquez becomes more settled. His heart rate and blood pressure return completely to normal. No more crying out. But he is still totally unconscious. He doesn't respond to me pinching his earlobe (another accepted check on conscious level). Apparently, my pinch is nowhere near as painful as whatever it is that makes him bellow.

'What happens now?' asks Ana in a matter-of-fact manner.

'We'll have to get him off the ship to a hospital where they can look after him in a proper intensive care unit. Have you got your insurance details – your travel insurance? We need to let your insurer know.' Ana leaves.

I bleep the captain.

'Captain, the patient is here in the hospital, the one from the Code Alpha. He's had a cardiac arrest. We've resuscitated him but he's unconscious. We need to get him off the ship to a hospital intensive care unit. We can't look after him here.'

'He's had a heart attack?'

'No. It was probably an abnormality of his heart rhythm. No sign of a heart attack.'

'So, are you sure you can't manage him on board? We're in Rio in two days.'

'Absolutely not. It would be an unacceptable risk to him. He needs specialised hospital care now.' I don't add 'and I don't know what the heck to do for him'.

'OK. I'll call the coast guard. Come up to the Bridge. You'll have to speak to the rescue service.'

On the end of the heavy, black ship-to-shore phone a woman speaks. 'Hello, I'm Doctor Klaas. What have you got for us?' Her voice sounds faint.

I start to summarise.

'Can you repeat? I can't hardly hear you!' Dr Klaas says, raising her voice.

I yell into the receiver, 'A sixty-five-year-old man sustained a cardiac arrest about an hour ago. We defibbed him and there was return of spontaneous circulation and breathing, but he remains unconscious.'

'What's the cause?' Dr Klaas shouts back.

'I suspect a cardiac arrhythmia, because he's been having fainting episodes. No sign of MI on his ECG.'

'Is he in sinus rhythm now?'

'Yes.'

'What are you treating him with?'

'IV fluids, oxygen, and morphine.'

'OK. We're on our way. About forty-five minutes.'

'They'll be here in forty-five minutes,' I shout at Captain Strom, handing him the phone.

I run down to the Medical Centre as casually as I can without causing alarm and type the referral letter. 'The helicopter's coming for Mr Marquez in forty-five minutes,' I announce to anyone who cares to listen.

'I've spoken to the insurance company,' says Liz. 'They just need a copy of your letter, then I'll let them know about the medical evac. I'll tell housekeeping to get their cabin packed up. Coralie!'

Coralie comes in from the resuscitation ward. 'What?'

'Is Mrs Marquez in with you?' Liz asks.

'Yes. Why?'

'Listen. Tell her that she and her husband are going to be taken off by helicopter in forty-five minutes.'

'Righto. She'll have to go up to the cabin to get their valuables – and settle her bill. Have you got their bill?'

'No, I'm doing it now. Wait and I'll give you it... hang on... hang on... here.' Liz waves it in Coralie's direction.

The stretcher team transfer our patient with intravenous drip and portable oxygen to the stretcher. He is to be transported to the aft deck through the Ocean Lounge to meet the helicopter. There is nothing else for it but to carry him through the lounge, out of the double doors at the rear and onto the deck.

It is gone eleven p.m. and the evening cabaret is still in progress. The orchestra plays, and the tenor, Baron Wild, is belting out *For Once in My Life*, the Stevie Wonder hit. The stretcher team, Liz and I enter the lounge, escorting our patient through the dimly lit area to one side, bending double, trying not to obscure the passengers' view of the stage. The tenor falters slightly on hearing our muttered cautions to bejewelled spectators to mind their shoes as we push by between the seats and tables. Mr Marquez emits one of his groans, making heads turn. I feel for the morphine ampoule and syringe in my pocket.

Emerging to dazzling spotlights illuminating the deck, a team of four firemen are standing each side of the deck in yellow high-viz jackets, trousers, gloves and helmets, with water-hoses unreeled, ready and pointing at the deck. No helipad here.

The stretcher team transfer Mr Marquez from our canvas

stretcher to a solid plastic bath-shaped one and strap him in tightly. His oxygen is removed. He groans more loudly. I give him half an ampoule of morphine through his intravenous line to last the flight, shouting in his ear, 'Mr Marquez. You're going to leave the ship on a helicopter. You're going to hospital.' No response. If he is having an out-of-body experience, even this solid reality will seem like a bizarre dream.

The sound of the helicopter blades grows louder. The ship slows. The helicopter comes into view, lights flashing. Like a loudly chattering UFO, it holds its stationary position immediately above the deck, travelling at the same speed as the ship. The night is velvet black. No moon. The ship rolls. If a propeller blade catches the ship's rigging, the helicopter will crash to the deck in an explosive molten fireball.

On a spindle of rope a slender woman in a fawn uniform descends in a standing position, like an elongated spider or a twirling trapeze artist, and steps nimbly onto the deck. The helicopter's blades, ten metres overhead, thunder, creating a hurricane of air. I brace my body, hold her arm tightly and shout in her ear, while our hair flaps about our faces.

'Dr Klaas?'

'Yes, Katerina!'

I bellow the updated medical summary at her, with a hoarsening voice.

Katerina signals to the UFO. A heavy metal clip lowers down on a line swinging in the agitated air. Katerina attaches a long rope to it. She lashes the clip to the centre point on the stretcher's straps, waving her arm in a circle above her head as a sign that it is ready to ascend. Slowly our unconscious patient in his plastic bath is winched up in the air, rotating and swaying in the down-draft like a chrysalis on a web, while Katerina steadies the attached rope. A man leans precariously far out from the side of the helicopter and levers the stretcher into the open hatch. A minute later our empty stretcher is lowered back to the deck.

Katerina unhooks the bath-like container, which is removed by the stretcher team, and holds the hook in her hand. The Marquezes' luggage has been lashed together as one large item. Katerina attaches the bags and signals. Dangling and twirling, up it swings, to be swallowed by the snarling machine.

Next a harness descends. Katerina puts her arm round Ana's shoulders and helps her into the harness. Then she attaches herself face to face with Ana for the two of them to be winched up together. The thin-looking rope with its suspended conjoined twins twists and turns until they reach the open door of the helicopter. Does Ana give a tiny wave as she and her web companion are man-handled in? The hatch door snaps shut. The helicopter is enveloped by the night's black infinity and silence.

The fire crews, stretcher team and deck-hands pack away equipment. The officers drift off. No debriefing.

I catch what sounds like a waterfall and shouting behind me and look round. Hundreds of passengers who have gathered on the upper decks are looking down, clapping and cheering. I want to burst into tears of relief but bite my lip and give a small regal wave. I guess I should have pulled my shirt over my face and skidded along the deck on my knees.

***

I find Tom in the Pool Bar. He gives me a long, tight hug. 'You were *terrific*.' Some of the passengers are looking at me, smiling and nodding.

I shake my head, aware of something new to feel guilty about. Here I am in this five-star floating hotel, specialising in diseases of the rich, an opulentologist. One elderly man becomes ill in the middle of the ocean and is saved by a flying medical service costing $25,000 per rescue, while women are dying in labour in Africa for want of basic road transport to a maternity unit.

Calculating my donation to Maternity Africa to redress this imbalance, I take the bubbly that Tom places in my hand.

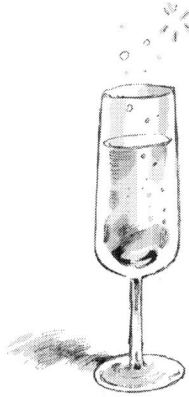

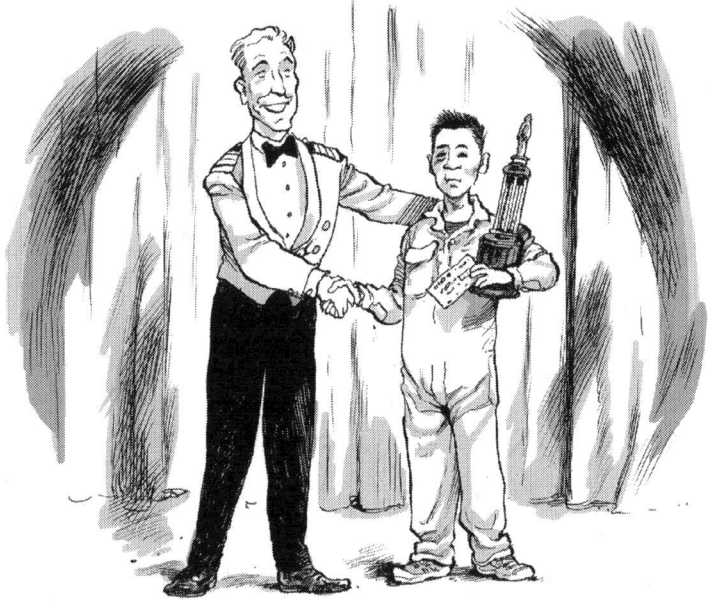

Day 18

Anjan

What is it about being at sea that makes passengers' legs swell?

There are two more leg-swelling cases in surgery with no obvious cause. From my extensive research of six patients, I deduce that it must be due to Taylor's Syndrome – a mechanism whereby the jolting, shuddering, rolling and pitching of the ship, aided by gravity, encourages fluid to pool in the feet and legs. Like shaking down an old mercury thermometer. I decide to write it up in the *Lancet* when I get home. Eponymous at last.

Anjan comes in with the eye patch still over his right eye, looking very sorry for himself in a pristine white boiler-suit.

'Eyes too much pain. Can't see,' he says, shoulders drooping.

'Let me take a look.'

I inspect the front of his eyes, then the back of them with the ophthalmoscope. They are less bloodshot than the day before, although his right eye is tearing. Again, I instil the stinging anaesthetic drops, then the bright orange eye drops that show up corneal ulcers. This time there *are* several tiny ulcers on the right cornea. Tiny. Pin-pricks. Had they been there the day before and I'd missed them? Or had they developed overnight? I hold up the eye chart.

The result is one line better on the left side, two letters better on the right.

'I can't see,' he insists. 'I want to see special eye doctor. Send me to eye doctor,' he begs.

Did he sense my lack of confidence treating a condition new to me?

'Anjan, your eyes *are* improving. Normally they will get better after about three days.' I'd said a couple of days previously; now I was conveniently extending the recovery period. 'It's early days yet. The test shows your eyes are better today than yesterday. Give it time. If you have pain take the painkillers. I'll see you again tomorrow. OK?' I give him another sick note.

'No eye doctor?' Pressure.

'Not at the moment. The eye test shows they *have* improved from yesterday. Each day they should be better and better. Slowly. Slowly. See me tomorrow.'

I look up arc eye online. One of the treatments is anti-inflammatory eye drops. I also have to be alert to him developing an eye infection. Is he despondent because of the condition, because he is off work with nothing to do, because he is afraid of losing his job or his eyesight? With his poor command of English, I feel inhibited from trying to explore his concerns in depth.

'Have we got any anti-inflammatory eye drops, Liz?' I call out.

'Anti-inflamm' *eye* drops? No. What do you want them for?'

'Anjan – the man with arc eye. Apparently they help.'

'No, we don't stock them. But you can order them from the port agent tomorrow.'

'Good idea.' I print the prescription.

'Listen. There's no-one waiting now. Let's check the dangerous drugs while we have the chance.'

The Medical Centre had gone quiet. We take all the morphine, pethidine, diazepam and other addictive drugs out of the safe, count them and record the amounts in the dangerous drugs book.

Before leaving I finish writing up the end-of-cruise log, now resembling a medical encyclopaedia, hoping there will be no more dramas to add.

—⚓—

Tom and I wander past the buffet restaurant. Mr Plummer is walking round the luncheon food display next to Moll, heads together, conferring about the choices.

The formal dining room smells of curry. Mrs Plummer is with a man from the table-tennis set. I wonder if he knows her diagnosis. Would she have disclosed it to him? Should I warn him? Do some spontaneous contact tracing? I decide against it, in public. As we walk past, Mrs Plummer leans out from her table. 'How's the patient?'

'Which one?'

'The helicopter man. Is he alright?' Table-tennis man listens in.

'Oh, I haven't heard. He should be OK,' I say, satisfied for the sake of confidentiality that I don't have any more details.

So far, I haven't found out what happens to repatriated patients, even if I ask to be informed in the doctor-to-doctor referral letter. It would be so helpful for my medical education, which inevitably involves life-long learning, or, in the jargon: Continuing Professional Development.

⚓

Back in the cabin Tom is keen to tell me about Joyce, Pam and Derek's quiz companion, who'd moaned at the lunch table about there being too many foreigners in her home town of Stoke and how she felt comfortable on board because she was among 'her own people'. Steve, a passenger we hadn't met, and his wife, Jude, stood up to Joyce's racist remarks and Tom enthusiastically backed up the new couple. Joyce accused them all of being 'liberal do-gooders' and flounced out of the dining room. Meeting the first couple to share our 'liberal-do-gooder' views is a rare treat and despite there being only two days left, Tom arranges for us all to meet.

⚓

At the Captain's Cocktail Party, I stand in the split skirt in military order alongside the other officers, greeting passengers. Unlike the Chief Engineer and the Safety Officer, passengers who have been my patients greet me as though I am a long-lost relative.

Mr and Mrs Plummer walk in at a distance from each other, nod, then hurry on to find seats, where they will be served with bubbly and canapés.

Albert and Harold approach. 'Did you find yer 'usband?' Albert asks, shaking my hand.

'Oh, yes,' I smile. 'Unfortunately, I'm stuck with him now.' I put on a pained expression.

'Sorry I've been such a trouble to you, lass.' He keeps hold of my hand. I think of contagion.

'It was no trouble, Mr Armsure. That's my job. Just delighted to see you well.'

'Are you off tomorrer then?' He lets go.

'Well, the next day. And you?'

'We're flying back. I'm not lookin' for 'ard...'

'Albert!' Harold intervenes. 'Other folks are waiting t' talk t' doctor.'

'Sorry love. Anyway, thanks for everything...' Albert says, as Harold pulls at his dinner jacket sleeve.

I spot Mr Wayfield a few feet away, with his wife. His gaze is averted as he walks determinedly to one side. Suddenly he leaves his wife and comes up to me.

'Thanks for looking after me, Doctor, and thank the nurses too, will you?' He turns and walks back to his wife as she squeezes along a row, heading for a free seat and table.

A woman stands in front of me. She is tall and buxom with a chiselled brown face and such high cheekbones that they give the impression of a perpetual smile. Her grey hair is coiffed into multiple tight plaits elegantly laced to her scalp. Grasping my hand warmly she croons, 'I think you've been *marvellous. So* busy. I can't imagine how you've coped. I'm an anaesthetist – *was* – retired now.'

'Ah.' That explains the connection. 'Thank you. Where did you work?' I look into her brown eyes. We know things – things only doctors know. The communion of the medical tribe.

'Nottingham. That was full-on and the *hours*... I don't have to tell you. I *know* how it is. Mind you, it's all different now, European Working Time Directive and all that. Miles better. So good to see a woman doctor on board.' She smiles a brilliant white thirty-six-toothed smile.

'Lovely to meet you.' I draw my hand out of hers, morale boosted. All this hand-holding is very unsanitary.

She passes on as Alice and Pat come over in their finery. Alice with her delicate, petite figure looks angelic in a long pale blue dress made of a floaty material, on her head a neat silver fascinator. Pat, a step behind Alice, is by contrast in a black velvet top with a scarlet skirt and large golden earrings. Gypsy Rosalie.

'Are you alright now?' I ask Alice. This is starting to resemble a ward round, in which the patients move along to see the doctor, rather than the doctor passing from patient to patient.

'Yes. I'm sure I'm fine, thanks.' She wouldn't have told me if she wasn't.

'You're looking well, Pat.'

'Thanks to you. I like your outfit, very smart.' Goodness, the compliments were on a roll.

Next on the rolling ward round is a heavy-set man with a bald head and a trim white beard. His dinner suit and red cummerbund sit uneasily on his convoluted frame.

'Heard the one about Tom Jones?' He grins broadly.

After years of oral exams, I always feel uneasy if I am asked a question that I don't know the answer to.

'A man goes to his doctor and says, "Doc, I can't stop singing *The Green, Green Grass of Home*." The doctor says, "You've got Tom Jones syndrome." The man says, "Is it common?" Doctor says, "It's not unusual."' He laughs loudly, his twinkling eyes igniting mine. There's always one.

Eric, the Cruise Director, is on the stage with the microphone in his hand. 'Ladies and gentlemen, please put your hands together for the Master of *Sea Rainbow*, Captain Ivor Strom!'

Captain Strom steps on stage to a drum roll.

'Good evening, ladies and gentlemen.'

Murmurings of 'Good evening, Captain' trickle from the crowd.

'We are nearly at the end of our first leg. Luckily, we have three more legs for balance.'

Subdued chuckles.

'Many of you are a different colour from when you boarded. I see you've taken advantage of the especially good weather we've had along the way. We haven't been so lucky with the stomach upsets unfortunately, but now I'm pleased to say all the stomachs have settled. We also struck an unlucky patch when we ran low on water after Cape Verde and I'm very grateful for your cooperation at that time. Speaking of luck, you might not know that we sailors are actually very superstitious. It's unlucky to sail on a Friday, or on the first Monday in April, or the second Monday in August. Well, we certainly didn't do any of that. But we still shouldn't sail if we see anyone with red hair, flat feet or crossed eyes before we board. Maybe that's why our luck changed.'

Laughter.

'When we board, we have to put the right foot on first, then make sure there are no pigs, rabbits, priests or flowers on the vessel. That's where we went wrong,' he says looking round at the flower posies on the tables. 'But, seriously, altogether we've had a successful cruise with some very nice ports. I think you've all enjoyed it, haven't you?'

'Yes, we have. Yes,' came a mixture of shouts and murmurs.

'Of course, I couldn't have done it without the assistance of our wonderful crew.'

The audience cheer and clap loudly.

'So tonight, I'm delighted to give this month's crew prize to a young man from the deck department. He has shown enthusiasm for his work, goes out of his way to help others, has a good attitude to his fellow workers and his supervisors. I'd like you to welcome onto the stage Anjan Shakya.'

Anjan? Really? Does the Captain know that he hadn't worn his protective goggles, against regulations? Is this why Anjan is so fretful about the condition of his eyes? Did he think that a specialist would cure him in time for his award ceremony?

In the wings there is a movement of the red velvet curtains and a disembodied arm thrusts Anjan onto the stage. He walks without his eye patches and navigates his way to the captain gingerly, squinting in the bright lights. Captain Strom puts his arm around Anjan's shoulders, emphasising the discrepancy in their heights as well as in their social standing, reflecting the developed and the developing worlds.

'How are you, Anjan?' Captain Strom, says looking down at him.

'Fine, sir.' Anjan looks ahead.

'How do you like working on board?'

'I like it. Better than home, sir.' He smiles.

'Better than home? So where is your home?'

'Nepal, sir.'

There is a ripple of 'ahhs' and applause.

'Anjan, it's a pleasure to present you with this cheque and trophy, as the employee of the month. You have worked hard, helped others and fitted in well. Congratulations.'

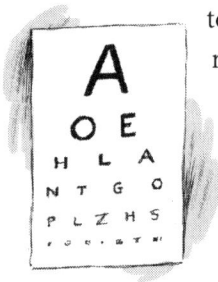

Captain Strom places the two items together into Anjan's left hand and holds his right hand in his own for several seconds while the photographer takes photos of the occasion. The room applauds loudly. Anjan walks to the red curtain, which is magically opened for him to pass through.

'Ladies and gentlemen, I can hear some stomachs rumbling now so I will not keep you any longer from your dinner. Thank you for travelling with us and I hope that we see you on our other voyages in the near future. Have a wonderful evening. Thank you.'

The orchestra strikes up Cliff Richard's *Congratulations* whilst the captain strides off the stage, handing the microphone to Eric.

'Let's have a big hand for the Master – Captain *Ivor Strom*.'

My calves feel stiff and my face aches from smiling. At least the sea is calm. I find Tom seated by a small table as passengers push past, heading for dinner.

He drains his champagne glass. It joins three other empties on the table. Not that I'm counting.

We have all just sat down to dinner in our finery when the photographer turns up.

'A photo of the table?' No-one answers.

'Yes – I mean, let's have a photo,' says Derek. He glances at the rest of us.

Mary and I echo him. 'Let's have a photo.'

Derek and Pam are placed behind the chairs that Tom and I occupy, so that all seven of us fit into the frame. The photographer tells us to say 'cheese'; then more photos are taken with our waiters, Manas and Danang.

Each couple submits to being photographed, leaning with heads together and smiling, and two are taken of Reg on his own. All will be displayed in the foyer. No obligation. I didn't think curmudgeonly Reg would have agreed to a photo, but he is in a cooperative frame of mind. Being a Formal Night there is free wine.

Everyone is upbeat and chatty. There is excitement in the air about reaching Rio and the anticipation of getting home two days later. Reginald has joined in with the bridge set and is beating other beginners. Jim is going to recite a Burns poem in the passenger talent contest. Derek and Pam are intent on photographing, then participating in, the special midnight feast on the theme of chocolate. We toast each other.

Suddenly there is a commotion behind me. I look up from my seafood jambalaya. Pam is saying, 'Ruth, there's a woman lying on the floor,' and nods past my shoulder. I think, *Someone should see to her.* Then I remember: it's me.

Looking round, I see Alice lying face forward on the carpet.

Pat is standing next to her. Mohan, the Maître d', crouches over Alice as one of the wine waiters comes up to me. 'Doctor, can you come? The lady fell off her chair. We called the nurse.'

I kneel next to Alice. She is conscious. 'You again,' I say. 'Trouble?'

'I'm alright. I'm alright, honestly. I must have fainted. Sorry, Doctor.' Alice starts to stir herself.

'I'm only teasing, Alice. Can you sit up?' I hold her arm.

'Yes, I think so.' She eases herself onto one elbow, blows a long breath through pursed lips and straightens up. She looks pale, her hair is out of place and the silver fascinator lays under her chair.

'Does anywhere hurt – arms, legs, chest?' I am squatting next to her.

Alice waggles her arms and moves her legs cautiously. 'No, nothing hurts. I'm alright. Honestly. So stupid.'

The passengers and officers at their delegated Formal Night tables are looking across the dining room at the stir, forks in the air. After a minute they resume eating and the buzz of conversation restarts. Liz appears with a wheelchair.

'Alice fainted and fell off her chair,' I tell Liz. I know Liz will understand that a simple faint rarely results in people falling off chairs. It will be something else. 'No sign of injury,' I add. 'FAST negative.'

In the Medical Centre I examine Alice. Liz does her ECG. It shows that Alice is in fast atrial fibrillation – her irregular heart rhythm racing at one hundred and eighty beats per minute. The fibrillating heart hasn't provided sufficiently strong beats to circulate the blood and oxygen effectively to her brain. So, it was essentially a kind of faint. Fortunately, there is no sign of heart failure. Not yet.

'Alice, it's your atrial fibrillation again. Your heart's going too fast for enough blood to get where it needs to go and that's made you faint. I'll give you something to slow and steady the beats. Have you ever taken digoxin before?' Alice is propped up on the resuscitation bed.

'No, but I've heard of it. Mm, yes. I think my mother used to take it. Is that possible? It must have been thirty or forty years ago, easily. Would that be right? I'm turning into my mother!'

'Yes, it's been around for donkey's years, at least fifty, but it's a good 'un. I can recommend it. You'll need to tell your GP when you get home. In fact, I'll write him a letter for you to take with you. We've got his details, haven't we?'

'My doctor's a she.'

I kick myself for making the sexist assumption I criticise in others. 'There is a charge for it. Nurse will tell you. Just ask on the way out.'

I hate all the charging, although I know the company couldn't possibly include medical services in the cost of the cruise. There'd be long queues. People would want second opinions on their GPs' diagnoses and third opinions on their specialists' views. Passengers would 'pop in' just in case they got sick, and want letters to change cabins or dining tables. They'd call in to sort out marital disputes or if they felt lonely.

I head straight to the Pool Bar, little knowing that there will be a revelation about the helicopter man, Mr Marquez. Steve and Jude, our new liberal-do-gooder acquaintances, are sitting with Tom, sipping drinks opposite Barbara and Lesley.

'How's your patient – the helicopter man?' asks Jude.

'He should be OK.' I cup my hands around a hot chocolate and brandy. Such a treat.

'His wife must be worried sick,' says Jude.

'She'll feel even more sick if he pulls through,' says Barbara. 'Her husband was an abuser. Bullied her, hit her, deprived her of things – everything.'

Jude gasps and puts her hand over her mouth.

'How do you know?' I ask.

'She told me last week,' says Barbara. 'Honestly. I think she would have been relieved if he'd died. She hated him. She confided in me because I got out of a situation like that with my first husband – years ago.'

A million what-ifs race through my mind. Should I have run so fast to the cabin? Should I have resuscitated him? Would I have tried so hard if I'd known about his domestic violence? What if doctors treated patients based on their moral worth? Who'd assess them on the morality meter? Didn't Médecins sans Frontières treat soldiers and victims according to their medical need regardless of the rights and wrongs of the conflict and which side they were on? What about the Hippocratic Oath? 'First do no harm.' Or in modern terms: 'Make the care of my patient my first concern.'

As for Ana's situation, I am reminded of one of my diabetic patients in Newham. An alcoholic, he had a gangrenous big toe unresponsive to antibiotics and the community nurse's dressings. At home he was a dictator. His wife and grown-up children couldn't speak to him unless spoken to. His behaviour would have been called 'coercive control' now. He stubbornly resisted being sent to hospital. Didn't want the control taken out of his hands. Semi-conscious, I finally sent him to the local hospital where he died a week later, aged fifty-three. I thought his wife would feel an enormous sense of relief and freedom. But afterwards she only ever appeared lost.

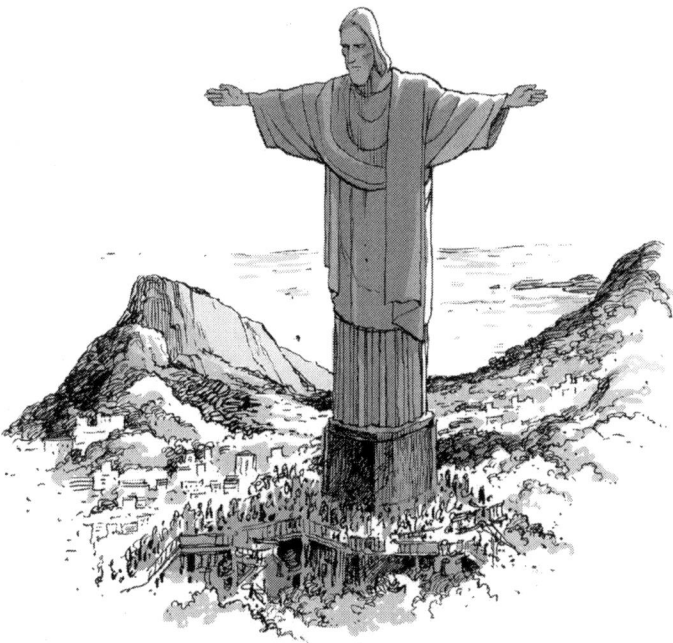

Day 20

Rio

Anjan is on his own in the waiting room.

'How are the eyes?' I ask as he follows me into the consulting room.

'Pain,' he says, screwing up his face and holding his hand over his right eye. The eye patch has gone. He is in civvies.

This time I can't see any of the tiny ulcers in the right eye that I'd noticed on the previous day, although they had been miniscule even then – less than half the size of a pin-head. The left eye is clear.

I wonder if my own eyesight is good enough to distinguish everything I need to see. Ophthalmoscope in hand, I look at the front of his eyes, then the back, but can't detect anything abnormal. Next the eye chart. The result is the same as the previous day, although he manages to name the letters more quickly and doesn't stumble. It seems like an improvement. I suspect he is exaggerating the pain, but I can't honestly be sure.

'Send me to special eye doctor. You do me a letter,' Anjan says, looking at me intently.

'I don't think it's necessary, Anjan. *Really*. Your eyes *are* improving. There's nothing more the eye doctor can do. We're getting you special drops today, from ashore. They'll help the pain and make your eyes better more quickly. Every day they're a bit better. That's what we expect.' When in doubt always use the royal plural. 'Come back this evening to get the drops. In the meantime, it's up to you to decide whether you can do your job or not. If you can do it without the pain interfering with your work, you can go back – only *use* goggles *every time* you're welding. But if you feel you can't do your job, I'll give you another sick note.'

I reassure myself that if the next doctor is concerned about Anjan's eyes he can always refer him at the following port in a couple of days' time.

'You've got another one,' Coralie says as she puts the notes down.

It's Mr Gardner, of the swollen legs.

'I thought I'd give you a chance to see me before you leave,' he says as he waddles in smiling.

'Very good. Come and sit down. How're you getting on?'

Have I asked him to see me again? He is paying for this so he must deem it of value.

'I think your pills are starting to work. My legs *are* improving.' He holds out a leg to show me.

'Good. And your diabetes? What are your test results?'

'About eight or nine with that extra tablet.' He looks all-round pleased.

I check his blood pressure and give him the reading.

Mr Gardner smiles at me in that admiring way I associate with men who take a fancy to me. Is that why he's here?

'Anyway, what does it mean, you know, the two numbers? My doctor's never said.'

I explain.

'It's clever, isn't it? What should mine be then?'

I tell him.

'Oh, I see.' He will have been told all this in the diabetic clinic. They give them information booklets too. 'So, what should my blood sugar be?' Delaying tactics.

'Eight to nine is quite acceptable. Do you need more pills?' I am finishing the consultation: next comes the prescription, then the door.

'No, I've got bucket-loads, thanks.'

'Good. Well, I hope you go on alright for the rest of the cruise, Mr Gardner. Enjoy the remainder of the trip.' I stand up.

'I hear you're a good dancer.' Oh dear. Here it comes.

'Well, I do enjoy it. And it's such good exercise too.' He is going to get the health promotion message while he is loitering with intent.

'I used to dance in my youth. That's where we met the ladies,' he muses, staying seated. 'Of course, I can't do the quickstep anymore, I get too out of breath, but I can still do the rumba. Would you give me the pleasure of a rumba?' There now. It is out.

'That would be very nice,' says Dr Charm-Itself. My heart sinks.

~⚓~

Tom and I stand on deck watching our passage into Rio harbour. There is no shiny thirty-five-piece brass band playing on the quay to welcome the ship, as there was in Yokohama in 1962 en route to Australia on P&O's S.S. *Strathmore* when I was fifteen. As soon as we'd docked, not one but two Miss Yokohamas in swirling kimonos came aboard with press photographers, to meet the captain and entertain the passengers with singing, dancing and playing of traditional instruments. Dad said that a Japanese prostitute wearing a bright blue outfit had boarded and, as she was permanently drunk, had enticed men into her cabin. Such a scandal. I wonder how Dad knew.

⚓

We watch Rio harbour looming up. Guanabara Bay forms a huge green indentation, curling round into the land, the massive statue of Christ the Redeemer overlooking the bay, with the lush, jagged mountains forming a dramatic backdrop.

Looking down, Tom and I spot a broad, snaking slick of rubbish wending its way past the ship from the inner harbour all the way out to sea. Plastic bags, bottles, wrappers and masses of indistinguishable, agglomerated flotsam and jetsam float past with dead fish entangled.

'Nice, isn't it? I had a really romantic image of coming into Rio,' says Tom.

'I'm taking no notice. I'm free for the day. Rio! Here we come!' I throw out my arms and fill my lungs to the brim with salty air.

⚓

Exit via the gift shops. I am immediately sucked into a sparkling store, seduced by the biggest, brightest, greenest emeralds I've ever seen. Rough, uncut chunks lay in a semi-circle in the dazzling showcase. Gorgeous and unusual: posh hippy.

'Those are six hundred pounds sterling. Columbian emeralds. Very good quality. Do you want to look?' asks a trim woman in a tight red outfit.

The prices must be means-tested, the fashion-model assistant calculating what customers can afford. No price tag.

'How much?' Tom is at my shoulder.

'Six hundred pounds.' I point to the emeralds. 'That doesn't seem too bad. They're huge. What do you think?' I know he likes to indulge me.

'If you want.'

'No. Come on. Let's do our art tour.'

At the bus stop the mix of people is different to those in Salvador. Many more whites, business types in suits; a few indigenous folk looking poor and preoccupied; black people offering shoe shines, cleaning the streets or sitting about. Portugal had ruled by skin colour when half of Brazil's population were slaves. Mr Tenerif-eh might have told us that in the 1856 census, the authorities listed seventeen distinct skin colours from 'white' to 'very dark'. The 'very dark' were relegated to the bottom of the social order and it looks as if that's where they've stayed.

As we step inside the bus, we are confronted by a revolving metal gate at the entrance to the seating area. It is released by inserting your fare into the slot. The door closes. Tom is just passing through the clacking turnstile when the bus lurches forward. Catapulted out the other side, he would have smashed his face on the window if he hadn't quickly clutched a handrail. Suddenly the driver brakes, throwing Tom backwards against the turnstile. He only manages to save his kidneys by tightening his grip on the pole with both hands. The whole scene looks so slapstick that a high-pressure guffaw tries to squeeze past my throat. But I dare not laugh. Tom looks shaken. Seeing the impending risk, I time my turnstile entry to coincide with the bus stopping at a red light. This it does only if the traffic in front stops. Vehicles jump the lights. Our driver, leaning imperatively over his steering wheel, overtakes other buses, hurtling along the wrong side of the road, causing oncoming traffic and pedestrians to swerve out of his way. Our formula-one bus stops with such whiplashing jolts that all we can do is to hang on white-knuckled, until Niterói Contemporary Art Museum looms up. Ashen-faced, we descend, grateful to have survived.

Tom turns to look at the mushroom-shaped museum.

'That's Oscar Niemeyer for you. Terrific modernist architect. Designed a lot of the buildings in Brasilia, the capital. He *loves* those curved lines. *Look at that.* Like...' he wags his head from side to side... 'a spaceship taking off.'

'Or landing... and right on the edge of the cliff.' I take Tom's hand as we lean over the rock face behind the gallery to look at the yellow beach a hundred feet below. There is a distasteful slick of debris all along the shoreline and a second ribbon of dried litter cast further up the sand. A thin black man picking his way through the rubbish has stopped to look at something in his hand. I start to feel responsible.

'Let's go inside,' Tom says, not given to sentiment.

None of the artwork is memorable, but the panorama forms the real work of art. The natural sweep of the giant horseshoe bay with its strange conical Sugarloaf Mountain looks like a dramatic nineteenth-century landscape masterpiece.

The rasp of cicadas and the rustle of brown lizards in the grass accompany our walk downhill into the suburb of Niterói. Tom likes to 'get the feel of a place', which to me always means wandering through parking lots behind supermarkets. I like to be purposeful.

Rat-traps are on sale but there are no long rubber gloves in the supermarket. Yet this is the country that was first to commercialise rubber, using indigenous slaves to produce it. Jesus, the galley hand with dermatitis, will just have to manage without them. No end of suffering for our Jesus.

'Let's eat here.' I am standing in front of a bright cafeteria with seating on a wooden deck under luxuriant trees, the breeze stirring their leaves.

Tom peers in. He is fussier about food than I am, wary of strange dishes and locations. As a sickly war-child he'd had to be coaxed to eat.

We load up our plates and take them to the cashier. She weighs the lot, plates and all. What an excellent idea. Let's face it – if all our restaurant food was weighed there might be a lot less obesity. The bill comes to twenty-eight reals, four pounds each. Tom orders a glass of pale local beer with oodles of ice and we eat in the shade feeling like royalty. What a marvellous thing this entire adventure is. Even the birds are singing.

Much of the beautiful art, music, writing and buildings in the world have been inspired by religion, so we atheists pay a visit to Christ the Redeemer. The bus takes us sedately to the base of Corcovado Mountain. Our ticket features Christ's Art Deco white face in close-up, European and solemn. The cable car, packed with a dozen tourists, looks too precarious to be carried by its narrow steel cables over cherry-red pylons. However, we pass high above thick palm and vine jungle to the seven-hundred-metre summit. Not a place for sufferers of acrophobia, a fear of heights.

'It's very Deco. When was it made?' Tom asks, craning his neck at the statue's face thirty-eight metres from its feet.

We look across to the white-roofed suburbs and out to sea, where solid clouds on the horizon look like snow-capped mountains.

I scrutinise the leaflet from the ticket office. '1931. No, actually it was started in 1922, but I don't know when the thing was first made – I mean the maquette.'

'Thing? That's highly blasphemous,' Tom teases.

'The face was sculpted by a Romanian sculptor – Leonida, not Leonardo, Gheorghe Leonida. Heard of him?'

'No.'

'Well, it says he's famous.' A challenge to Tom's B.A. Fine Arts.

'Obviously not famous enough. It's elegant though. I'm surprised I like it,' Tom says, head thrown back.

The odd contour of Sugarloaf Mountain rises above the bay to the west. It was named after the shape of the original loaves of sugar produced for export in slave times.

'He's been struck by lightning twice.' I giggle. 'Hand of God.'

'Well, that'll learn 'em.'

The café on the lower terrace offers the equivalent of Walls ice-cream, the ubiquitous dolce-de-leche (tooth-achingly sweet) caramel biscuits and hand-fried crisps. At least the coffee is Brazilian. We wobble our cups down the steps to a table near the edge of the terrace where the greenery of the mountain tumbles away.

Something rustles in the undergrowth. 'Look,' I whisper, 'look down there. *There.*' I point. 'See that bush on the left? See down the bottom near the trunk, just to the right. There's a big stripy lizard, really big. See?'

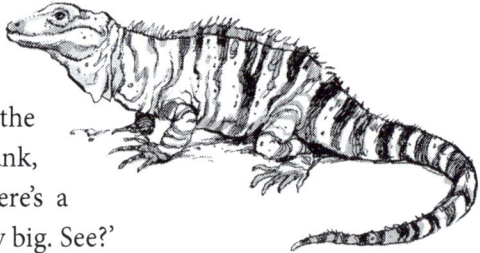

'Where?' Tom peers in the wrong direction.

'*There. Look.* Can't you see the trunk of that bush, the one with spiky leaves?'

'Yes.'

'Well, about six inches to the right of the trunk there's a bit of a clearing. Do you see?' We are both leaning forward, staring into the bush.

'Yes – oh, *yes.* It's *massive.* Powerful head. Fantastic stripes

– gold and black. Now *that's* a real work of art. Must be at least four foot long.' Tom leans further forward, his head almost in the bush.

'Well, two feet.'

'Three foot six.'

'Two foot six.'

'Looks like a kind of iguana. It must live up here eating leftover crisps and dolce-de-leche biscuits,' I say.

'We have to move. It's nearly three-thirty. You'll be *late* again. *We've got to pack.*'

I let myself into the empty Medical Centre. The cleaners have been round, the smell of chlorine reminding me of Ironmonger Row Baths, where I swim with friends in Hackney. I settle down to finalise my end-of-cruise report. The waiting room bell rings. *Blast.* Can't I just *get on*? Marion is standing with her finger on the buzzer.

'Marion. Come in.'

She follows silently and sits down.

'How did you get on with your scan?'

'They said it could be cancer.' Her face crumples and she starts to cry, tears rolling out of the corners of her eyes. I pull tissues out of the box and give them to her, briefly laying my hand on hers.

'Have you... got the report?' I ask.

'No. They said they'd send it to you.' She was choking back the tears now, mopping her face.

'Right. Let's have a look.' I open the e-mails. No e-mail. 'It looks like it hasn't arrived yet,' I say. 'Tell me what happened. What did they say exactly?'

'She put this thing inside me and she spent a long time

poking about and looking at the screen. Then she said there was a *mass* in the ovary. Lucky for me she spoke English. I asked her what it was. She said she couldn't tell for sure. I said, "Could it be cancer?", then she said… "It could."' Marion's eyes redden, her nose runs and she cries again, tugging in a sob.

'OK, so it might or might not be cancer. Well then, it's really important we get that report. I'll ring the hospital. Also, remember the blood test I left you a note about? That will give us important information. If that's normal, it's very unlikely to be anything cancerous.' 'Cancerous' sounds less like a cancer than 'cancer' does. 'But if both are suspicious, then you'd be better off in England getting it all sorted out. Leave it with me and I'll start chasing. As soon as I've got news, I'll let you know.'

I hear Coralie come in, noisily opening and closing drawers and thumping things down on the desk. I open the door and put my head round.

'I've got a patient with me, Coralie. Can you keep the noise down?'

She gives me an expression that seems to say, *'So?'*

Marion looks towards the door. 'It *is* confidential, isn't it? No-one else will know, will they?'

'It *is* within these walls, yes, but when you go ashore, you know that several departments have to be informed. But they wouldn't know what you're going for. I'll ring you as soon as I have something to tell you.'

'Coralie?' I shout round the door. 'Do you know which hospital Marion was sent to this morning?'

'It'll be Samaritan – *Samaritino*. What d'you want to know for?' Suddenly she is taking an interest.

'I have to chase up some results – they haven't sent them.'

'Sometimes we don't get results for a week or two.'

'A *week*! That's useless. I need to know today. Depending on the result we might have to repatriate her.'

'Repatriate Marion?'

'Well, yes, *maybe*. Is there a Portuguese-speaker on board who can translate?'

'Zack – the IT Officer.'

'Could you call him down right away?'

Zack is in his twenties with a pale, serious face and black-rimmed glasses. His hair is so brown, thick and shiny it could pass for a wig. 'I can't stay long. I'm supposed to be in the passenger IT room at five-thirty.' He was dressed in crumpled Junior Officer's cream trousers and jacket, with one stripe on each sleeve.

'I have to get some test results from the local hospital for a crew member. A scan result and a blood test. It's confidential, of course.'

He pushes his glasses up his nose.

I dial *Samaritino Hospital* and hand the phone to Zack. 'Ask to be put through to the blood test results department.' We wait. 'When you get through tell them it's the Medical Centre on *Sea Rainbow* and ask for the result of the Ca 125 blood test.' I write it down with Marion's name and date of birth on a post-it note and push it in front of him.

Zack starts speaking, listens, speaks again, then waits. 'She says we must speak to the patologia department. They're transferring…' He speaks at length. It sounds like a repeat of the whole story. 'He asks when it was done?'

'This morning.'

'*Esta manhã*,' says Zack. 'He says it's not through yet.'

'When will it be through?'

'Maybe one hour.'

'*Maybe*? Tell him we need it urgently this evening. Can he e-mail it to me as soon as he has it? Tell him to put you back to switch – we need the scan result.'

Zack says, 'Telefonista,' and holds on… and on. 'It's cut off.'

I ring back. It's engaged. How can a hospital be engaged?
I ring again. 'Ask to be put through to the scan department.'
Zack speaks... waits... speaks. 'What was the scan for?'
'A pelvic scan.'

'*Pélvico escandir*... She says I have to speak to the X-ray department. I'm going back to the switchboard.' The only bit I recognise is '*departamento radiografia*.'

It is gone five-thirty.

Zack is talking, then listening. 'She says she sent the result at three o'clock – to the e-mail address on the top of the letter.'

'That's reception. Give her mine. And ask her to send the report now.'

I e-mail the reception manager asking her to look for any e-mails from *Samaritino Hospital*, to send them on to me, then delete them. A few seconds later the e-mail drops into my inbox.

The text refers to a '*sólido e cístico*' something in the ovary, five by four centimetres. '*Cisto dermoide*' is the report's conclusion. There it is – exactly the same terminology as in English: a dermoid cyst – normally containing a mixture of benign tissues. But I need the Ca 125 blood test to be more confident that there isn't a malignant element to the cyst. It is a tiny possibility. I check the time. If the Ca 125 was to be sent through an hour after Zack's call, it will be due in half an hour.

I ring Marion. 'I've chased the hospital. They're sending the results through in about half an hour. I'll call you as soon as they arrive.' I don't want to give her the scan result until I've received the blood test result as well. I want the full picture.

The Ca 125 arrives. It is normal. My neck stops aching.

Marion sits down heavily in the chair. Her eyelids are red-rimmed and puffy. I hold the scan result in my hand and go over the results.

'*Oh, God. It's not cancer then?* Oh God! Thank heaven.' Tears of relief trickle down her cheeks. More tissues. 'Oh God... But you say it's a sort of sac? What's inside the sac? How did it get there? How do I get rid of it?'

'It's a slightly odd story – but a few of the cells in your ovary didn't ever develop into proper adult ovary cells – they stayed as infant cells, which can turn into any tissue, so they've just decided to grow into extra hair, or fatty cells, or even teeth. All sorts. It's probably been there for ages – years, getting a little bigger until it's big enough to press on something and give you pain. But the thing is that the cyst can sometimes twist and cut off its own blood supply, or bleed – not commonly, but occasionally, so you'd be better off getting home to have it taken out.'

'You mean an operation?' Marion straightens her back.

'Yes. But they might be able to do it by keyhole. It will be up to the gynaecologist.'

'Do I have to be repatriated? I'd rather stay on. Honestly. My contract finishes in ten days' time. Can't I stay?'

'Do you want to?'

'The company won't find a replacement at such short notice and everything is set up for the new stock arriving, the end of cruise sales… stock-taking… all next week. Then my replacement will be here anyway.' She is herself again, efficient, in charge.

When Marion leaves, I ring Dr Wallis.

'Emergency?' There is noise in the background, a kind of muffled railway station announcement.

'No, not really. It's a crew member who's been having pelvic pain. The scan shows a dermoid cyst in the right ovary. Ca 125 normal. Her contract is up in ten days. Would it be OK for her to stay on till the end of her contract?'

'I see no reason why not. Dermoid cyst, you say? Nothing much can happen in ten days.'

'It can tort, or bleed.'

'Ah yes. You're the gynaecologist. What do *you* think?'

'It's not a big risk. I couldn't quantify it though.'

'If she signs a disclaimer, she can stay on. One piece of intelligence for you: I'll see you at lunchtime tomorrow.'

'What d'you mean?'

'I'm at Heathrow now, about to board. I like to see the new doctor at the end of their first cruise, just to make sure everything is alright.'

———⚓———

At dinner Mary says, 'It would be so lovely to keep in touch. This is our address.' She passes me a carefully cut slip of paper. 'Ye must come and see us whenever you're in Scotland, so you must.'

'Thank you, Mary. Shall I give you mine?' I say, fervently hoping that I won't need to socialise with our companions again. Over the course of the cruise, as I have got to know them better, I have developed a level of concern about them as individuals, but rather like patients whom I've seen several times. We have too little in common to develop firm friendships.

'Oh, yes please. On the back of this.' She turns over an address slip and gives me a pen. 'Although we dinna get to London so much. Too hectic and noisy for us.' That's lucky.

The chances of us being in Scotland are close to zero. It is hard enough to get Tom anywhere outside the M25 London orbital motorway.

'Did ye see Christ the Redeemer? Wasn't he just marvellous? It felt so peaceful up there… as if I was close to heaven,' Mary says.

'A little exaggeration, Mary,' says John.

'No-o. I really did feel very peaceful there next to him. I can't explain it. It just was.'

'We liked it, didn't we, Derek?' says Pam.

'Yes, I wasn't expecting him to be *so huge. Enormous.* Dominates the whole bay,' says Derek.

We exchange goodbyes, handshakes and unexpected hugs. The farewells feel oddly temporary. Chances are that we'll all bump into each other numerous times along corridors and in lounges before we finally disembark in reverse order of cabin numbers the next day, the top-most cabins down to the lowest deck. Thanks and tips in small brown envelopes are dispensed to our dedicated waiters, Manas and Danang.

~⚓~

As we walk up to the Pool Bar for the last time, I ask Tom about Reg and Barbara. 'They're an item. Turns out she lives near Colchester and they both like golf. So, they're going to meet up.'

'*Well, I never.* Good old Reg.'

Lee is playing *Sweet Home Chicago*, his foot tapping the piano pedal, head nodding: a fast jive. Tom and I sit down to let our meals settle. The dance hosts and the usual crowd must have been at the farewell show because the room is almost empty. Ron is sitting at the bar with his drinking pal. He comes over when he sees Tom. 'Have you heard that Man U beat Chelsea two-one?'

'*Sod it,*' exclaims Tom. The two revel in their final analysis of Arsenal's chances and of the relative merits of being on ship or shore during the height of the football season.

Lee sings *Honesty* by Billy Joel. A Why Dance. Just right for a busy digestion. We press ourselves snugly against each other and sway to the music, moving as little as need be. It is so good to be close after the long daily separations. Warm and welded together, I can breathe in Tom's scent as we shift languidly from foot to foot. Then comes *Goodbye Norma Jean* by Elton John. A rumba, well suited to pancreatic activity. I feel a tap on my shoulder. 'May I?' Mr Gardner asks Tom.

Despite big feet and swollen legs, Mr Gardner's rumba is a delight. He certainly has the rhythm. He concentrates on the three basic rumba steps while leading me into complicated sashays around him. No close hold. The rumba isn't like that. At its most fiery it's a passionate tussle of attraction and repulsion. We coolly display our fan, hockey-stick, New Yorker, open hip twist, alemana, rope spin and Cuban rocks while we talk about the journey home. Such an unexpected pleasure.

Mr Gardner leads me by the hand back to my seat.

'Shall we go?' Tom says.

'Let's just see what the next dance is.' I don't want to leave. Once we go out of the door there will be no more dancing until a rare family wedding or barmitzvah. *I Feel Good is* an energetic number by James Brown. Our uninhibited 'wiggle' is Tom's favourite. We lock our gaze and revolve around each other until the very last note.

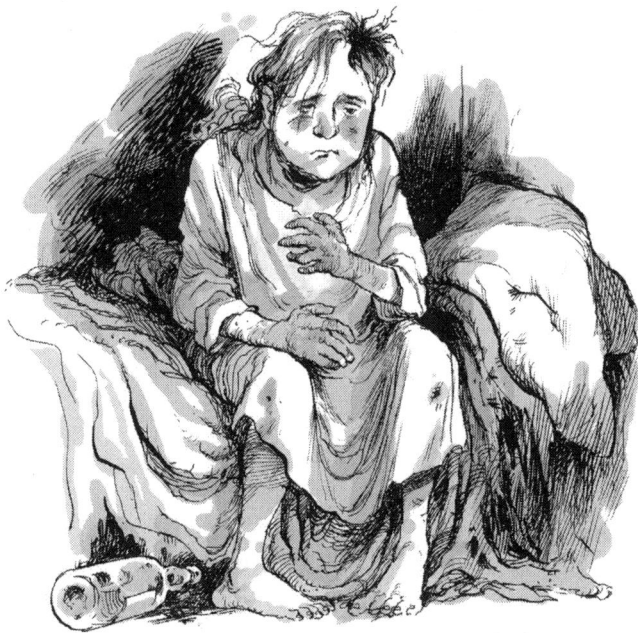

Day 21

Coralie

Smoke. The corridor reeks of smoke. Cigarettes? Burning paper in a waste bin? I step up my pace. A thin grey haze is curling out from under one of the cabin doors at the far end of the passage. The tannoy hisses.

'Code Bravo, Code Bravo, Code Bravo, cabin three-two-four – starboard side. Repeat, Code Bravo – cabin three-two-four – starboard side.' The sensitive Bridge equipment will have registered fire from the smoke detector in the cabin. Isn't three-two-four one of the nurses' cabins? My chest feels hollow. I run.

Two firefighters in high-viz jackets are advancing from the far end. They stop in the smoky fog, hoses in hands. A third one is near the open cabin door and a fourth in the doorway.

Coralie's voice croaks. 'I'm orright! I'm orright!' accompanied by coughing. 'No more water,' I think she says. As I press forward,

I can see Liz running towards me from the opposite end of the corridor.

An acrid smell seeps from Coralie's room. She is sitting on the edge of the bed, head in red swollen hands, coughing, her fringe singed. The pillow and the top of the bedding are scorched and sodden; so is one side of Coralie's nightgown. Liz shouts to the stretcher team to bring the stretcher into the cabin.

'I can walk,' Coralie rasps. The side of her face and her arm are burnt. Her eyes are bloodshot and streaming.

'No, you *can't*,' Liz insists.

'Don't put me on the stretcher,' Coralie coughs out.

'Just get on it, Coralie,' I say. She doesn't look at me but allows herself to be helped onto the canvas, flinching when the oxygen mask is fitted.

One of the stretcher team's feet clinks against something under the bunk. He pulls out an empty vodka bottle and puts it in the bin. As the team move into the passageway, I notice the short man with glasses standing there again. He must be some sort of ghoul.

In the Medical Centre we clean and dress Coralie's first- and second-degree burns (red skin and blisters). Fortunately, they are not deep. We put up an intravenous line and give her painkillers.

'What on earth happened?' Liz asks.

'Must have been a ciggie. S'pose I fell asleep. Bugger of a cruise. Worst bloody cruise ever.' Coralie's breath smells of alcohol. Not last night's.

'You'll be off the ship and home soon,' I say. Am I reassuring her or myself?

Liz arranges the repatriation, going in and out of the ward to check details with Coralie. I order the ambulance then ring Coralie's mother, trying not to make a drama out of the incident. After all, she must be well aware of her daughter's foibles, and besides, Coralie won't be left with permanent scars. But it might be a career-ending incident. She is an addict to nicotine and alcohol. A sign of psychological distress. Self-medication. She needs help. Maybe she'll get it, if she grabs the chance. Soon she'll be SEP – Someone Else's Problem.

I leave and change into a flouncy multicoloured travel skirt and black top, set off by radioactive orange plastic earrings and necklace. It gives me the delightful feeling of being an uncaged bird about to flap its wings and fly. An antidote to being confined with medical emergencies. I hurry down to Dayap, arms heavy with used uniforms, and say my goodbyes to him and the labouring laundry crew in their underwater cavern.

Back in the ward I approach Coralie. Angry as I am with her, both her behaviour and this calamity, *she* is the one losing out and suffering, so I turn on my compassion button to setting number one and touch her arm. 'I'm sorry it's turned out like this,' I say, and I am. Coralie looks at me but says nothing. Her eyes fill.

Liz and I see Coralie off the ship and into the ambulance on the dockside. Liz gives her a tentative hug. The ambulance door shuts.

Liz starts stock-taking. I send off the voyage's medical log to the Captain, the Chief Officer, the Cruise Director, Reception Manager, five sister ships and Dr Wallis. All the medical personnel in the fleet like to learn from each other's experiences. At least we haven't had to deal with three cardiac arrests in the first hour of *our* cruise – which the medical team on one of the sister ships had faced. With a shudder I imagine having to dash from one crisis to the next, leaving a third of a nurse to cope with the outcome of each critical incident. Then ringing the relatives, the insurance companies… I'm not going to think about it.

The phone rings. Liz calls out, 'Lisa wants you in Accounts for your seaman's book and pay. That should be the good bit, what with all the noros. You'll be laughing.'

'I'll laugh when I can draw breath,' I say.

The accounts office is near the Bridge. My seaman's book has been signed personally by Captain Strom under the details of the voyage. Lisa, the accounts clerk, stony-faced, counts out my wages behind her grill. Four hundred and twenty-seven pounds and forty-three pence. The notes are folded carefully and eased into a brown envelope with the coins. Cash in a brown envelope. It feels illicit. Inside there is a printout of passengers' details and my half of their bills. The other half goes to the company. I scan the list. And again, more closely. This doesn't look right. Four hundred pounds is all very nice, very nice indeed, but hardly recompense for a woman of my calibre being flogged near to death for twenty days, no time to even cut my toenails. Suddenly it seems like a pittance. Twenty pounds a day. I sit in the card room on the Bridge deck examining the statement. There are names of patients I've treated missing. At least a dozen noros aren't even mentioned. Mr Marquez has been charged for two consultations and medication, but not for his hospital treatment. Then I see that two phone calls to Dr Wallis's number in the UK have been deducted from my wages. Twelve pounds and forty-five pence. I go back to Accounts. Lisa hears my complaints impassively. 'It's only what the nurses send us. We don't decide. If the nurses don't give us the information, we can't pay you. You must ask them.'

'But what about these phone calls?'

'If you dial straight out from your office it goes onto your account. If the call is Medical Centre business it has to be cleared through reception.' The accounts' officer looks weary. It's her busiest day and I am holding up the queue.

'Well, how am I supposed to know?' My voice is harsh. Other crew waiting in line for their pay are staring at me, muttering to each other and shifting from foot to foot. I suppose they think that there is nothing for a doctor to complain about – a highly paid, privileged Senior Officer.

'It's for the nurses to say.'

The nurses. The nurses.

'Liz. I've seen Lisa for my pay but honestly, it's a fraction of what it should be,' I say. 'There are loads of noros missing from the printout, and Mr Marquez was not even billed for his hospital stay. That's three hundred pounds a day for a start, isn't it? What's going on?' I am standing over Liz at the desk.

Now the one who didn't want to get involved with the filthy lucre and didn't like patients being charged is agitating about not charging patients enough. It is the principle of the matter, obviously.

'Coralie was doing the noro billing,' Liz says. 'But I can check Mr Marquez's account. I might have forgotten to add the hospital charges.'

'Will you print me out the noro log, Liz? I'll check it against my statement.'

Just then Dr Wallis appears, smiling. 'Morning all. Good cruise?'

'Busy,' says Liz.

'We had the noro outbreak,' I enjoy reminding him, 'half a dozen emergencies and a helicopter lift-off.'

'Ah, yes. Still, at least you had the second doctor.' He rests his hand on the desk.

'What second doctor?' I ask.

'John. John Lancaster, the surgeon. He was on as back-up if you needed him.' Dr Wallis looks at me as though this was common knowledge.

'I didn't know we had another doctor.'

'Didn't he introduce himself? Short chap with glasses.' Dr Wallis glances at me then looks away.

'Wait a minute. That sounds like the man who hung around when the emergency codes were called.'

'He should have come down to see you. I'll have a word with him if he's still on board. Never mind. You'll be home tomorrow.'

'Well, I have another problem, Dr Wallis.' I was now doubly aggrieved. 'My pay hasn't been calculated properly. There's a lot missing: noro patients and hospital stays,' I say.

'Ah,' he says, nodding. 'Still, as long as you've had *fun*, that's the main thing. Has it been *fun*?'

'Mm… I suppose so-o.' My vocal cords feel strangled.

'That's capital then,' he pronounces. 'So, we'll see you aboard again. Very good. Is Coralie about?'

'You haven't heard… sit down.'

Liz and I tell Dr Wallis about Coralie's fire and her repatriation.

'I see… dear, dear me. Well, good thing you're getting another nurse. Vicki will be here tomorrow. She's on her way.'

'Vicki? Oh, that's *great*. I love Vicki.' Liz's eyes lit up.

'Very good then,' says Dr Wallis, standing up. 'Capital work, girls,' and he turns on his heels, practically clicking them together.

Liz and I sit adding the missing fees to the system. In Accounts a second brown envelope is handed over.

At reception I stop to say goodbye to Angel and her colleagues. Mr Wayfield stands in front of me at the desk waving a piece of paper. 'There's *two pounds* on my bill for water. Those bottles were *free*. I shouldn't have to *pay*. You could just take them from the trolley on your way ashore!'

'Sorry, sir. The water for guests on tour is fifty pence a bottle. That's why there is two pounds on your bill, sir.'

'Nobody said it cost fifty pee. If I'd have been told, I could have taken water from our tap. We should have been told.'

'But nobody else thought the water was free, sir.'

'That's nothing to do with me. I wasn't told I had to pay, so *I'm not paying.*' Mr Wayfield's voice had become strident. He stood anchored to the carpet.

'Just a moment, sir, I'll speak to my manager.' Angel disappears behind the door at the side of reception and returns after a minute.

'We can take the two pounds off your bill, sir.'

'So, when are you going to do it?'

'We've done it, sir.'

Mr Wayfield leaves. I look at Angel, pursing my lips and raising my eyebrows. 'Thank you for looking after Lorenz, for sending him to a specialist,' Angel says.

'Oh, you know Lorenz?'

'He's my husband. We married last year.'

'That's wonderful. Well, I expect the skin specialist will get him on the right track. Maybe see you and Lorenz next time.'

'I hope so. Take care, Doc.'

'Where the hell have you been?' Tom demands. He is standing with our cases at the airport shuttle bus stop on the quay.

I tell Tom about Coralie's revenge and Dr Wallis's rescue plan.

'Anyway, I'm never doing *that* job again, I can tell you. That's the first and last time. *Bloody slavery,*' I say.

Tom casts me a look. 'Slavery? *Really?*'

'Well, alright – not in chains, not indentured labour, but hard graft, with insufficient reward. That sort of slavery.'

'But you've always *loved* that sort of slavery.' We laugh.

Two days later Dad rings from Australia eager for news. He was thrilled that I'd landed the job.

'How was the cruise, darling? Was it *wonderful*?'
I hesitate. 'Yes Dad, it was wonderful.'

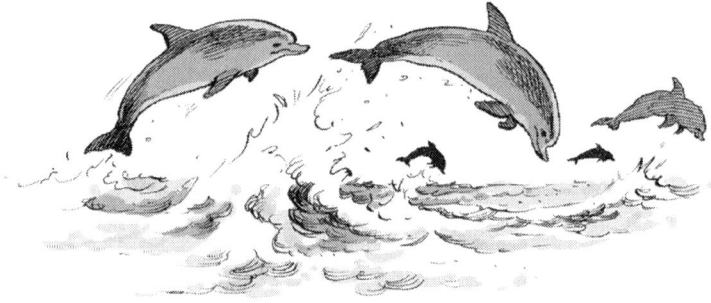

Food Consumed

Eggs – 41,400

Ice cream – 3,125 lt

Cheese – 890 kg

Butter – 795 kg (portions – 60,000)

Cream – 2,250 lt

Flour – 3,750 kg

Milk – 5,700 lt

Soup – 375 lt

Fish – 4,383 kg

Poultry – 3,130 kg

Pork – 2,547 kg

Vegetables – 6 tonnes

Beef – 2,711 kg

Potatoes – 4,375 kg

Lamb – 1,590 kg

Fruit – 4 tonnes

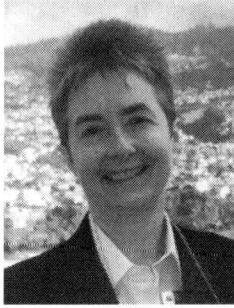

Ruth Taylor's ocean voyages began aged two sailing to Australia with her family as a Ten Pound Pom. Sea travel became her passion. As a 21-year-old ship's nurse she was determined to retrain as a doctor. From her busy East London GP-practice she returned to working on ships regularly during holidays accompanied by her husband, Tom.

ABOUT THE ILLUSTRATOR

David Parkins was born in Brighton but spent most of his early life in Lincolnshire. In 2022, after 16 years in Canada, he returned to the UK with his family and a couple of Canadian cats.

Over a long career, he has illustrated many children's picture books and fiction titles for publishers in the UK, US, Canada and France. He worked for the UK comics *The Beano* and *The Dandy* for many years, drawing, among other characters, *Dennis the Menace* and *Desperate Dan*.

His editorial work includes illustrations for magazines including *Nature*, *The Economist* and *Bloomberg Businessweek*. He also creates political cartoons, which have appeared in *The Guardian*, *The Observer*, and, in Canada, *The Toronto Star* and *The Globe and Mail*.

Since September 2022 he has been drawing a daily editorial cartoon for *The Globe and Mail*, Monday to Friday, fitting his other work in where he can. Sometimes it's a bit of a tight fit. Despite his venerable age, retirement isn't on the horizon. Not yet.

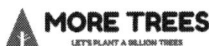